Advan

brother-in-law

push

"We have finally come to understand that birth and death are best understood in their proper context as social events—ones that ought to, at their best, involve others. This book, taking on Murray Enkin's long-established views on both, celebrates these ideas in an articulate and deeply touching way. A must-read after the depths of isolation caused by the recent pandemic."

—SHOLOM GLOUBERMAN, Philosopher in Residence at Baycrest Health Sciences Centre in Toronto, Ontario Canada, Founder of Patients Canada, and author of *The Mechanical Patient: Finding a More Human Model of Health*

"A thoughtful exploration and comparison of life's most important passages (birth and death) full of insight and practical suggestions. I recommend this book to healthcare professionals and anyone else who has been born, lives, or might someday die! I grinned, I wept, and then I went back and made notes!"

—JO OWENS, author of *Another Kind of Paradise*

"My mother was dying. I sat beside her hospital bed, knowing it was for the last time. A young nurse came to say goodbye. She was going on maternity leave and my mom had been a favourite patient. Mom looked up. Slowly and with difficulty, she placed a trembling hand on her swelling tummy and said, 'One comes in and one goes out.' At an unsettling time for all of us, it was a warm, enchanting moment. It was also the truth. As one of us leaves the planet, we make space for the next arrival: a time for emotion, celebration, and profound change. Susan Boron has studied the many similarities in this wondrous cycle. Through both clinical and personal observation, she takes the reader through the trauma of goodbye

May our recently birthed friendship continue to grow!

and the thrill of hello with kindness and candour. For health professionals and the rest of us as well, Bookends is a well-researched, thought-provoking and comforting read.

I have known Susan's family for many years. I will be forever grateful to Susan's dad, Dr. Murray Enkin, for helping me begin my own career. Murray died recently. We celebrated his rich life as best we could, uplifted in knowing that he changed obstetrics forever and created opportunities for others who now take his place. The cycle continues. One comes in and one goes out....and each event is a miracle."

—LYNN JOHNSTON, author of *For Better For Worse* (the cartoon series)

"With warmth, wisdom, and compassion, and after more than four decades of caring for her patients, Dr. Susan Boron reflects on the poignant drama and inevitability of birth and death and the surprising parallels between them."

—JACALYN DUFFIN, MD, PhD, author of
History of Medicine: A Scandalously Short Introduction

Bookends

A Family Doctor

Explores Birth, Death, and

Tokothanatology

———

Susan Boron, MD

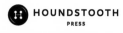

HOUNDSTOOTH
PRESS

Hardcover ISBN: 978-1-5445-3131-1
Paperback ISBN: 978-1-5445-3130-4
Ebook ISBN: 978-1-5445-3132-8

Author photograph © Meagan Hayward Photography

In memory of Doug Boron and Murray Enkin.

No doubt, the two strongest influences in my life.

Contents

Foreword
by Murray Enkin[1]

Thursday, March 4, 2021

THERE IS NOTHING THAT COULD BE MORE FLATTERING TO A father than to be asked by his daughter to write a fore word to her own book, a more eloquent book than he could have possibly written. a book by his own daughter, who had put into practice a corollary to the aphorism that he tried to live by. "If you didn't write it, you didn't do it". The corollary is that if you didn't do it, you shouldn't write it.

My field was maternity care. I came into that field by a series of accidents. I wanted to be a chemist, but my father said "OK, be a chemist, but get your MD first." So I got my MD, but on the way got upset by the way that I perceived doctors and nurses were treating pregnant women, and especially women who were giving birth. At least two...

Introduction

I had seen birth and death but had thought they were different.
—T.S. Eliot

Know that birth and death are the crest and trough of one wave.
—Laurence Galian

I TIPTOE INTO THE HOUSE IN THE WEE HOURS OF THE NIGHT, careful not to wake the sleeping household. I pour myself a glass of wine and sit in the dark in my comfortable chair contemplating the night's events, the lives forever changed. I am emotionally charged as I review my role in the whole thing: what I could have done better, what went as planned. I think about my patient and their loved ones.

I can't tell you how many times I practiced this little ritual after a delivery, remembering the adrenaline rush of having a baby slip out of a mother's body and into my hands, warm, wet, and crying lustily.

And how many nights I spent going over the final moments of a patient who had slipped over into death, the tears shed by the family, the sense of loss, the sadness.

For over forty years, my general practice involved patients across the full spectrum of health and illness. The office visits, the tests, the procedures: these were the mainstay of my day-to-day work. It was always fun and challenging to see the vast variety of diagnoses and diseases that came through my door. But I came to realize my most satisfying work was at the bookends of life—the births or the deaths of my patients. And I realized that, in many ways, those bookends were the same kind of practice.

Wait. Delivering babies and palliative care the same thing? What am I talking about? Birth is a happy event, cute, cuddly babies, excited parents, joy joy joy. And palliative care is morbid, sad, a failure of what medicine has to offer. It is grief, pain, and demanding, unhappy families. But both are complex, intense events that require expertise and compassion on the part of the caregiver. There are many common threads in the professional care we provide, and this one is a concept in its own right. This is tokothanatology.

Tokos is the Greek word for childbirth. *Thanatos* is the Greek word for death. And *-ology* means the study of, or the discipline of studying, as in geology, psychology, or epidemiology.

So the study of childbirth and care for the dying is called tokothanatology. It's a real thing. Or it will be for you by the time you have finished reading this book.

This is not a textbook of obstetrics or of palliative care medicine. I promise not to bog you down with scientific jargon, medication doses, or therapeutic plans. There are better sources for those, and believe me, it is vital to have the medical knowledge and skill along with the touchy-feely things I will talk about. To provide one aspect of care without the other makes for poor medicine.

Think about it. As a doctor, these are the times in the life cycle of our patients that we have little control over. Both of these life-altering events are going to happen regardless of any intervention. That baby is going to be born whether we are there or not. And that person is eventually going to die whether we interfere or not. But we can walk alongside our patients and help make their experiences better physically, emotionally, and spiritually.

My patients and colleagues heard me say many times that I was going to write a book about this someday: the idea that there are so many parallels between what we provide in obstetrics and in palliative care. My thoughts percolated over the years, and I filed them away while I was busy living my life and doing my work. Then COVID came along, and I was isolated at home with just my dog. Travel plans were cancelled, social expectations were put on hold, and well, it was someday. So here we are.

This book will share some of my thoughts and experiences with the hope of helping doctors and other care providers increase their level of comfort in dealing with the dying, using the skills they already employ in their care for pregnant women and young families. My premise is that the principles of care we provide at the beginning of life are mirrored at the end of life. Just as significant, and just as gratifying. I would like to help you see the parallels in the many aspects of birth and birthing, and death and dying, to help you enhance your practice and enrich your life in the process.

CHAPTER 1

Why I Am the One to Write This Book

The two moments are much alike: birth and death are made of the same fabric.
—Isabel Allende

Tokothanatology: During my career in medicine, I learned that people facing terminal illness need many of the same things that women giving birth need.

M Y FATHER IS A DELIVERY MAN. Actually, he was an obstetrician, and a rather renowned one at that. But I heard him say "I'm off to do a delivery" many times, so I told my Grade I classmates that's what he did.

Murray W. Enkin—MD FRCSC FACOG LLD (hon) D (hon) CM to the rest of the world, Daddy to me—was passionate about his work in maternal care. He talked about his love of women—pregnant women in particular. He said he made a commitment to himself very early on to do something about the way women in labour were treated. He vowed to change the status quo of the doctor being in charge and the woman having no involvement other than just being there. He was an early advocate of Dr. Grantly Dick-Read's philosophy that a woman's mental and emotional involvement in the delivery of her child improved the experience, and of Dr. Fernand

Lamaze's method for reducing pain in labour without medication by teaching exercises and breathing techniques.

Even before my father finished his internship in the late 1940s, he was teaching prenatal classes to his patients. His plan had been to become a general practitioner who did good obstetrics, but after a few years in rural Saskatchewan, he moved our family to New York to study and specialize in obstetrics and gynecology. Then we moved to Hamilton, Ontario, a city with a large immigrant population. Daddy saw the need for an Italian-speaking obstetrician in the city, so he hired a tutor, and he and Mommy learned Italian at our dining room table. My sister, Nomi, four or five at the time, became quite fluent in the language. Sitting near that table, I learned only two things in Italian. One was how to count to ten, *"uno duo tre..."* The other was how to say *"spingi"* ("push"). Hmm.

After my father attended an international conference in Paris in 1962, featuring Dr. Lamaze's principles of psychoprophylaxis in obstetrics, he and my mother began teaching prenatal classes in our basement, promoting prepared childbirth as an alternative way of giving birth. I remember pregnant ladies streaming into our home with their husbands and their pillows for their weekly classes. I sometimes came home from school to find a pregnant couple in our living room. Daddy would invite his patients to our home for part of their labour—because we had a bathtub, and the hospital didn't; and because my mother would give the women something to eat, and the hospital wouldn't. It was a quick trip across the road when it was time to deliver.

Daddy was the first obstetrician in Canada to have fathers in the delivery room. On one occasion, he dressed a father up in scrubs, gown, mask, and shoe covers and had him watch the birth of his child silently. Only after the birth did Daddy reveal what he had done to the hospital administration.

My father was the first to deliver women in the labour room instead of moving to the sterile delivery suites. He challenged many of the standard procedures of obstetrical care of the time, such as episiotomies, shaving, and enemas. And later, as birth became even more medicalized, he questioned the routine use of technology such as fetal heart monitors for low-risk deliveries. Routine procedures, in his view, often became empty rituals, without good evidence to support their continued use. He would sometimes sleep on the floor outside of his patient's hospital room, to protect her from the "routines" done to women in labour. No wonder he missed so many family dinners!

He went on to do extensive teaching and writing, promoting family-centred maternity care and prepared childbirth. He worked closely with many of the leaders of childbirth education, such as Elisabeth Bing,[2] Sheila Kitzinger,[3] Suzanne Arms,[4] Doris Haire,[5] and others. Some of these women became his good friends and visited with our family. I remember staying with Elisabeth Bing in New York as a teenager one New Year's Eve. Daddy must have been working with her, or maybe it was just a social visit. Her apartment was decorated with a huge collection of pre-Columbian figurines, mostly pregnant women, women giving birth, and fertility statues. After experiencing Times Square at midnight, we got to sleep in the room with her amazing sculptures.

My father wrote forewords to these women's books, supporting the concepts they promoted. He was influential in organizations such as ASPO (the American Society for Psychoprophylaxis in Obstetrics) and ICEA (the International Childbirth Education Association), and he edited and wrote for journals related to their causes.

In collaboration with Marc Keirse and Iain Chalmers, and with my mother doing all the bibliographic work, my father did

---

2   See *Six Practical Lessons for an Easier Childbirth* (New York: Bantam, 1967) and *Moving through Pregnancy: The Complete Exercise Guide for Today's Woman* (Indianapolis: The Bobbs-Merrill Co., 1975).

3   See *The Complete Book of Pregnancy and Childbirth* (London: Dorling Kindersley, Ltd., 1980), *Rediscovering Birth* (Boston: Little, Brown and Company, 2000), and *Birth Your Way* (London: Dorling Kindersley, Ltd., 2002).

4   See *Immaculate Deception: A New Look at Women and Childbirth in America* (Boston: Houghton Mifflin, 1975).

5   See *The Cultural Warping of Childbirth: Improving the Outcome of Pregnancy through Science* (London: Academy Publications, 2014).

a thorough study of all of the literature on pregnancy and childbirth, reviewing it for the quality of research and the evidence on effectiveness. They classified practices by those that improved outcomes, those that caused more harm than good, and those that had no effect on outcomes. They wrote and edited *Effectiveness and Satisfaction in Antenatal Care* in 1982,6 and then *Effective Care in Pregnancy and Childbirth* (ECPC), which was published in 1989[7] and later morphed into the Cochrane Collaboration,[8] now one of the most prestigious platforms for assessing and presenting all medical research and guidelines. There is a vast section on palliative care in the Cochrane now, as well.[9]

The group realized that the robust ECPC textbook was not accessible to the average birth attendant: the midwife in Africa, for example, or the family doctor in rural Saskatchewan. So they later wrote the bestselling *Guide to Effective Care in Pregnancy and Childbirth*,[10] a small, inexpensive summary of the ECPC and all the results— positive, negative, and neutral.

My mother, Eleanor Enkin, was a birth photographer. Many couples hired her to take photographs of their labour, delivery, and family moments. Some of her photographs grace various books about pregnancy and were used in my father's lectures and her own.

My father's advocacy for pregnant women and for the best of all possible experiences in childbearing carried over into the rest of his life's philosophy. Personal choice was always the most important principle of care for him. As he aged, he talked about the same

6   Iain Chalmers and Murray Enkin, *Effectiveness and Satisfaction in Antenatal Care* (London: William Heinemann Medical Books, 1982).

7   Iain Chalmers, Murray Enkin, and Marc J. N. C. Keirse, eds., *Effective Care in Pregnancy and Childbirth* (Oxford: Oxford University Press, 1989).

8   "About Us," Cochrane, accessed March 27, 2022, https://www.cochrane.org/about-us.

9   "Palliative Care Database," Cochrane, accessed March 27, 2022, https://papas.cochrane.org/palliative-care-database.

10   Murray Enkin, Marc J. N. C. Keirse, and Iain Chalmers, *A Guide to Effective Care in Pregnancy and Childbirth* (Oxford: Oxford University Press, 1989).

principle at the end of life. He was fascinated by the palliative care work my husband, Doug, and I did. He embraced choice, education, and excellence in care for the dying. He was a strong advocate for the "death with dignity" concept, promoting the right of a person to die in the way and at the time of their choosing. Let's just say that we had many heated discussions about this subject over the years. He coined the word *tokothanatology* to describe the study of birth and death and talked about it often. (I still claim the idea was mine.)

So I grew up in a home where pregnancy, deliveries, prenatal care, and patient choice were routine parts of the dinner conversation. Didn't everyone?

My childhood answer to that universal question, "What are you going to be when you grow up?" was "a Mommy with eleven children—or a Mad Scientist." Instead, I applied to medical school. Like most medical students, I wanted to go into each speciality as I did the rotation in that field. In particular, I loved obstetrics, geriatrics, and psychiatry. I remember, in a verbal exam during my OB rotation, being asked about the progress of a delivery and describing the whole thing, step by step, using my hands to demonstrate. I heard one of the examiners whisper to the other that I was a natural. And then I had a rotation in family medicine. I knew right away that was my fit—I wanted to be the doctor who could care for the whole person, to see them as a complex sum of all their parts, mind and body.

I did a family medicine residency, got married in the process, and then practiced in Hamilton for a couple of years before choosing a practice in the small town of Kincardine, on the shore of Lake Huron—mostly because the delivery room in their hospital had a big window facing out onto the lake, and I thought that was just wonderful.

I was well trained in the obstetrical practices of the time, so when I began delivering babies, I followed all the standard routines. But with my father's ideas planted firmly in my head and the cockiness (or naivety) of youth, I pushed the limits and started to ignore a lot of the rules. At the time, there was a fairly rigid set of procedures for childbirth. At the onset of labour, the woman was admitted to hospital, examined and prepped (i.e., her pubic area was shaved and she was given an enema), and put to bed. Once labour was well established, the woman would be encouraged to get her epidural. Her husband might have been allowed in the labour room but was invited to leave for any examinations or procedures. When it was time to deliver, she was transferred by stretcher to the delivery room and placed on a narrow bed with her legs up in stirrups and sterile drapes covering her body. Her husband was relegated to the waiting room to await the blessed event. The cartoon image of fathers smoking, pacing in waiting rooms, ready to give out cigars was very real.

An episiotomy was standard, and forceps were used often to "facilitate" the delivery. After the delivery, the baby was examined, cleaned up, given needles and eye drops, shown to the mother briefly, and then moved to the nursery, lined up with all the other babies. At that point, the father was usually let in to see his wife, and to see his baby through the glass window of the nursery. Babies were brought in to the mothers at regular times to be nursed or bottle-fed. The nurses gave sugar water as the first feeding and cared for the babies in the nursery. Mom would be moved yet again to a postpartum room to stay in the hospital for about five days. Her other children were not allowed in to visit but could wave from the hospital grounds below.

I remember that part very well. When my youngest sister, Jane, was born, I was eight. I saw my mother in a tiny window, waving at us. I met the baby for the first time on the way home from the hospital. My other sister, Nomi, two years younger than me, had been delivered by our father in a small town in Saskatchewan; but now we were in the big city, so my father, an obstetrician himself, was not allowed into the delivery room.

From the very start of my practice, I preferred to do deliveries in the labour room and allowed the woman a lot of freedom of choice in her labour. I encouraged prenatal classes, birth plans, and the Lamaze method of pain control over epidural anaesthetic.

I never saw myself as a pioneer, but simply as a proponent of the right way to practice obstetrics.

When I moved to a smaller centre, I assumed my methods would be easily accepted. There were no anaesthetists to do epidurals—and rural communities were closer to the natural order of things, right? Well, yes and no. Rural hospitals run without specialists. Basically, the whole medical staff is involved in every department, so things are a bit less structured. But all the doctors and nurses were trained in the cities and followed the same guidelines, so it took some convincing before they accepted my "radical" ways.

I resisted the idea of having to move my patient, at the very time when she felt overwhelming sensations of pushing, onto a narrow stretcher in the delivery room, and instead encouraged women to remain in the same bed they had laboured in to deliver their babies.

I gave my patients a choice, unheard of in our small hospital, on whether they would have the shave and enema routine, and most of them (of course) declined. One of the OB nurses approached me, saying the nurses had concerns about forgoing enemas on admission. She said the women were likely to pass some stool when they started pushing. I asked if the mothers were more distressed by this possibility or by the enema itself. The answer was clear. The fact that the vagina and perineum are not actually sterile at any rate helped to reassure her. It was sufficient to simply wipe away the poop with a clean cloth. Our hospital policy changed.

With practice, I learned how to help a woman control her pushing and to protect her perineum with olive oil and warm cloths, so I very rarely did an episiotomy. I actually took part in a study that showed that a small tear at delivery was better than cutting the perineum, allowing for easier healing and less long-term discomfort. I started teaching Lamaze-type classes at the hospital. Over time, we introduced rooming-in rather than keeping babies in separate nurseries. And we switched to birthing beds and birthing rooms rather than labour rooms and delivery suites. We encouraged families to bring in their music—it was on tapes back then. Later, I would realize music was just as beneficial in the dying person's hospital room.

By the way, I was the first female doctor the town had known, so there were many other challenges, too—but that's another story.

Thirty years later, I moved my practice to another small town: Hanover, Ontario. One of the reasons for the move was that they were still delivering babies, and Kincardine had abandoned their OB department seven years previously. Along with a full general practice, I was back doing my beloved obstetrical care. According to hospital policy, I had to be supervised for the first few deliveries. After so many years of doing obstetrics, I shouldn't have been nervous at all, but I was. When it came time to attend a birth at Hanover Hospital, another doctor was in the room to watch me. I sat down on the bed with my patient, and suddenly I was in the zone. Nothing mattered but the progress of this baby entering the world, his mother, her perineum, the baby's heartbeat. "Little push, little push, pant, pant pant, that's it, little push, little push, I see the baby's hair, OK that contraction's over, take a big cleansing breath and smile. It's over. OK here's the next one, push, push, little push, pant pant pant, gentle push, OK there's the baby's head, yes it will burn a little bit, OK, there are the shoulders, that's lovely, and one push, swoosh, here's your son! Here Daddy, would you like to cut the cord? Right there, that's good, now we will put your baby on your tummy. Yes, you can touch him! He's beautiful! Keep him warm with this blanket while we deliver the placenta." The miracle was back. I loved it!

Years later, as Hanover's obstetrical service was at risk of closing because many women were choosing to go to the city to deliver so they could have the option of an epidural, several of our doctors set up an on-call system for epidurals. The number of women choosing to deliver locally increased dramatically, and there was once again a viable OB department, with over one hundred deliveries a year and an active teaching programme.

MY EDUCATION DURING MEDICAL SCHOOL about death and dying was very limited. Training consisted solely of a twenty-minute film based on Elisabeth Kübler-Ross's book *On Death and Dying*,[11] in which she described five emotional stages of dying: denial, anger, bargaining, depression, and acceptance. And this was at the beginning of my first year of medical school, long before we had any contact with real patients, let alone severely ill people.

In Kincardine, through the years, my practice was aging along with me. Fewer of my patients were having babies; more were developing heart disease and cancer. I saw a gap in the care I was providing for these people. I learned about a new idea called palliative care, and I was intrigued. I began studying and learning about this new branch of medicine and looked for some funding from the hospital to start a palliative care programme.

Getting seed funding was a challenge—the administrator at the time felt it wasn't necessary. "But people have always died in our hospital!" was his explanation. We were finally able to set up some training in pain management and care for the dying, as well as a volunteer visitor programme as an added layer of support. I read books and took many courses on palliative care, which introduced the ideas of education, choice, autonomy, involvement of the family, the importance of excellent symptom control, and the value of dealing with the spiritual and emotional health of the dying person along with the physical. These sounded a lot like the principles I was using in the obstetrical part of my practice. Hmmm.

I found myself on a hospital committee charged with developing a palliative care programme. And at the same time, I remember an epiphany I experienced. Let me share it with you.

I was doing a shift in Emergency, which usually involved twisted ankles, sore throats, sports injuries, and the occasional motor vehicle accident. And a lot of heart-related problems. I was well trained. I had done the ACLS (Acute Cardiac Life Support) and ATLS

---

11   Elisabeth Kübler-Ross, *On Death and Dying: What the Dying Have to Teach Doctors, Nurses, Clergy and Their Own Families* (New York: Scribner, 1969).

(Acute Trauma Life Support) courses, which encourage the use of an algorithm for emergency treatment. We are taught a common pathway so that things go smoothly with a cardiac arrest, and we all follow the same protocol.

A woman had been brought in by ambulance. She had collapsed at home; the family had started doing CPR. The ambulance arrived in short order, and the paramedics carried on the resuscitation all the way into the ER.

A quick look at her monitor showed an irregular heartbeat and no blood pressure. She was not responsive. The algorithm goes through the medications to give and when to give an electric shock to the person's heart. As the physician in charge, I went through all the steps, and with each step, my patient's heart responded perfectly. It began to beat regularly for a while, and then reverted to an arrhythmia. We continued CPR, we gave the next medication, and her heart responded perfectly. And then deteriorated again. Again I ordered the proper treatment, and her heart responded favourably.

But she didn't wake up. We continued the steps, the treatments, and each time, her heart only did what it was supposed to do for a period of time.

In the meantime, the air ambulance arrived, and arrangements were made to transfer her to London, our tertiary centre. The paramedics carried on with the resuscitative efforts, loaded her onto the helicopter, and flew off with her.

Only then, I turned around and saw her family. They had watched while we heroically tried to save this lovely lady's life. They watched from the corner of the room, hoping and praying for their mother, wife, centre of their family, to wake up and see them there. We were so busy trying to save her life that there was no time to let them see her, or touch her, or say goodbye.

She died in the helicopter en route to the city.

Any of my readers with cardiac knowledge will recognize that my patient had electromechanical dissociation. The electricity in her heart responded as it should have to the medications I ordered for her. But the muscle in her heart had been damaged enough that it didn't work in response to the electrical impulses, so there was no circulation, and no oxygen reaching her brain. She was actually dead before she got in the helicopter, likely even before she got to our hospital.

The loving family were under the impression she would get better, that we would cure her. And in fact, as the doctors and nurses moved through all the right steps, we probably believed that, too. It's what we were trained to do, after all. There was no time to reflect or think.

But looking back, if I had taken a moment to really think about it, the signs were there that her life was gone. Her blood pressure did not improve; her level of consciousness did not improve. I could have accepted that and had her family approach her bed, say they loved her, say goodbye, shed their tears, and let her go.

Something about this scenario felt very wrong. She did not deserve to die hooked up to machines, up in the air and away from all of those she loved. And they did not deserve to live with the unresolved grief of never being able to say goodbye.

That day, I swore to myself that I would never forget the person I was treating. That I would think before I jumped into a rote kind of resuscitation without considering whether it would be the right thing to do.

PEOPLE SAID MY HUSBAND, DOUG, had a "palliative" soul. He was always acutely aware of people around him who were dealing with loss. In fact, some of our dates would start with a visit to someone who had lost a loved one. It's just who he was. When I asked him to attend a palliative care course I was teaching to give me some pointers on my teaching style, I should not have been surprised that he signed up as a palliative care volunteer at our hospital. "You need some men! Dying men don't need sweet little old ladies to hold their hands; they need someone who can relate to their anger, their needs."

And I was not surprised when the hospital asked him to take over the Palliative Care programme a year later. He coordinated a team of trained volunteers who supported dying patients. He won the respect of the professionals and the community. Referrals came from the physicians, nurses, clergy, and patients and families themselves. Doug and the palliative care team followed patients throughout their illness and death and into the bereavement period, no matter if they were in the hospital, at home, in a long-term care facility, or even had been sent to a city hospital for treatment. His programme was fairly unique. There were palliative care services in other small hospitals, and in the cities, but by and large with more of a medical orientation.

Doug developed an on-call system for sudden death support. This was not the usual palliative care concept, but it was well received. Whenever there was a sudden death or a gravely ill person brought into our ER, we automatically called in one of the volunteers. They introduced themselves and offered to be there with the family, to sit with them while a resuscitation was going on, to serve as communication liaison between the medical staff and family, or to bring coffee and cookies to the family while they waited. Often these volunteers would carry on supporting the families after a death occurred. If they were not welcomed, they simply withdrew. That rarely happened. A volunteer could also be called in when a death occurred in the community. The really difficult ones—the suicides, the children—Doug frequently dealt with himself.

His education was by no means medical, and in many ways, that was an advantage. He had studied philosophy in university (a sure path to the job market, he used to say!) and attended art school after that. He worked as an auto machinist, artist, art teacher, farmer, and maple syrup producer.

Doug read voraciously about palliative care and became well versed in the medical aspects of terminal illness, pain, and symptom control. I think we were the only husband-and-wife team to attend advanced palliative care courses together. He would call on me to prescribe pain medications, to do medical assessments and consultations, and to be the liaison with the other physicians as required. Whatever it took to get what his patients needed.

Today, palliative care is taught in medical schools, and most hospitals and communities have palliative programmes. They are often part of a hospice, with outreach into the community, with doctors and nurses on call, doing home visits as well as hospital consultations. These teams are now the experts in pain and symptom management in the terminally ill, and they offer support to the families. I think the programme we had in Kincardine all those years ago offered comprehensive holistic care, during the dying time and afterward.

On our twenty-fifth wedding anniversary, I delivered a baby; Doug was with a young woman as she died. So we cancelled our plans to go away overnight and felt the fullness of our life's work instead. The next day, we were both back working at the hospital. I was called to the Quiet Room, I thought to talk to the family of one of my patients. Doug was paged to the Quiet Room, too, and we arrived at the same time. The family of his patient had heard about our anniversary and had brought in takeout Chinese, set up a table and candles, and wished us a happy anniversary. The best celebration ever!

And then Doug got sick. Very sick. I learned what it was to be a family member/caregiver rather than a doctor/caregiver. Totally different. I knew the system; I knew how to access all the things my patients needed, but when it came to Doug's needs, and mine, I was as lost as anyone else. I learned that dealing with a serious illness was all-encompassing and overwhelming. I felt alone and helpless.

I looked critically at all the things I had taken for granted, like the idea that patients heard what I was saying, that they could make decisions about options while I was discussing them, that they would feel my empathy and they would trust me. None of it happened as easily as I had thought. I had no idea what we needed or how to access it, and no idea what to ask when confronted with, "Do you have any questions?"

In some ways, it is a disadvantage being in a medical family. Your doctor assumes you—the patient—know what your spouse knows, and so you are not treated or talked to as thoroughly. It seemed to fall on me to figure out what was going on. I have to say, Doug had an excellent family doctor who did everything he could. By then, Doug had retired from palliative care, and we had moved away from the community where he was well known, so he did not have a working relationship with the doctors. And besides, he was stubborn and had become distrustful of doctors (except me) (or maybe me as well). There was very little medical science had to offer Doug at that point. We spent a lot of time at our remote, off-the-grid cottage, until the cold weather pushed us back home. Eventually, I arranged some extra help at home, although I was solely responsible most of the time.

In the course of his illness, Doug was my only priority. I cut my workload and then took a complete leave of absence. His illness was a lot more aggressive than we were led to believe.

After he died, I knew things would be totally different but thought I could get back into my practice without too much difficulty. It took a long time, and I never did have the same commitment or the same confidence. After about a year, I was ready to retire.

In the meantime, my mother died. Mommy's death was a good one. She was ninety-three years old and had advancing dementia. My parents were still in their own home, with some help. Daddy did her hair every day; he would kiss her, and she would always smile and kiss back. Whenever he got a bit frustrated with her, he would ask, "What's the password?" and she would purse her lips for a kiss. Very sweet.

Then she deteriorated and needed total care. Her caregiver quickly realized what was happening and asked the family to call the palliative care team. Victoria, BC, has a very robust, quite wonderful programme of community palliative care. They arrived within hours, and another layer of caregivers were introduced. My dad stayed right with my mom. He wrote in her obituary, "I kissed her with each breath and then there were no more, and I kissed her again."

For the rest of that day, the whole family gathered around and told stories about her life and the wonderful things she did for all of us. It really doesn't get any better than that.

So, as you can see, I have spent a good deal of my life immersed in the milieu of birthing/obstetrics and dying/palliative care. And I realize that a lot of my colleagues see these two aspects of family medicine as beyond their scope of practice. Delivering babies is a joyful but demanding, unpredictable endeavor. And dealing with the dying is also challenging. With every birth I attended, I felt the miracle; and with every death, the privilege of being part of the journey.

I would like to see family doctors and other caregivers become more comfortable and more involved in working with patients at both ends of life.

Before we look at how to provide the best care, I'd like to look back a bit at how modern obstetrics and modern palliative care have evolved.

CHAPTER 2

A History of Obstetrics and Palliative Care

Technique has taken over the whole of civilization.
Death, procreation, birth all submit to technical efficiency and systemization.
—Jacques Ellul

It is as natural to die as it is to be born.
—Francis Bacon

Tokothanatology: Pioneers in medicine have brought about many lifesaving measures and better outcomes for childbirth and severe illness. But there has been an ongoing battle between scientific advancement and patient-focused care.

Obstetrics

Throughout history, pregnancy and birth were treated simply as normal events, not medical procedures. Traditionally, there would be a woman in the community, or sometimes a family member, who would act as a midwife to support the pregnant woman and to aid in the safe delivery of the baby. Childbirth was not thought of as an illness but merely as a part of a woman's life. In most cultures, men were kept away from birth altogether.

Maternal and infant deaths were just part of the landscape; childbirth was a dangerous undertaking. One in three women died during childbearing age in the middle ages.[12] And the chances of a child dying before his first birthday were as high as 25–40 percent until the middle of the twentieth century.[13] But babies were born, and many lived, grew up, and had babies themselves.

Traditional ways to support women during pregnancy and birth have been passed down through the generations. There are many depictions of births in ancient art and texts, often showing women giving birth in an upright position, squatting or sitting. However, we really know very little about birth practices throughout history. Because common people did not write about their experiences, our only records are about the "very important" people (mostly royalty), and mostly written by men. And men were banned from the birthing arena almost completely. By the middle ages in Europe, male doctors were called in by midwives only when there were problems during deliveries, and when there was money or rank to justify the use of these esteemed men. The intentions behind these practices were usually good: to make childbirth less dangerous for the mother and the child, and ultimately to make it less painful. It is likely, of course, that there were some issues of control at play rather than pure benevolence, as the following story shows.

A family of surgeons, the Chamberlens, introduced a special tool in the early 1600s to aid in complicated deliveries. Prior to that, when there were problems, the baby had to be extracted by means of hooks and other tools, always at the expense of the child—and often the mother, as well. Not pretty.

Dr. Chamberlen was able to successfully deliver a stuck baby without the death of the child or the mother, by means of a new device called forceps. His family kept their invention a secret, even

---

12   Sarah Bryson, "Childbirth in Medieval and Tudor Times," The Tudor Society, accessed April 20, 2022, https://www.tudorsociety.com/childbirth-in-medieval -and-tudor-times-by-sarah-bryson/.

13   Max Roser, "Mortality in the Past—Around Half Died as Children," Our World in Data (blog), June 11, 2019, https://ourworldindata.org/child-mortality-in-the-past.

going to the extent of blindfolding the mother, bringing the device into the birthing room in special gilded boxes, and applying the forceps from under blankets. The Chamberlen family published a paper describing only one half of the forceps apparatus, making it impossible to use properly. (The key to the use of forceps was to slip one side in, then the other, attach them around the skull, and then pull, applying pressure equally.) The Chamberlens were able to keep the secret of forceps for many years and benefited financially from their monopoly. When the secret leaked out in the 1730s, other physicians made some modifications, but the original concept has survived basically as first devised.[14] Forceps are still in use today, although less commonly. The application of forceps required an episiotomy. Until relatively recently, especially in North America, an anaesthetized mother, a large episiotomy, and a forceps delivery was the norm, and the accepted right way to deliver a baby.

Gradually the medical profession—i.e., men—took over the birthing process, marking the start of modern obstetrics. Up until then, childbirth was usually in the hands of a midwife, and doctors or "male midwives," as they were called, were only brought in when things were not going well. Gradually, the medical profession's role in birthing became a fashion and then standard practice. In North America, especially, midwifery became suspect, "unprofessional," backward.

Birth was moved to hospitals and overseen by doctors. General practitioners did most of the deliveries, calling on specialists only where there were complications or high-risk pregnancies. Over time, in many communities, obstetricians began doing more and more of the normal deliveries, as they still do today.

Surgical delivery, or caesarean section as a mode of delivery, is mentioned in many early documents, from Chinese etchings

---

14   "Secrets! The Curious History of the Chamberlen Forceps," Case Western Reserve University, College of Arts and Science, Dittrick Medical History Center, October 26, 2017, https://artsci.case.edu/dittrick/2016/03/28/secrets-the-curious-history-of-the-chamberlen-forcep; Sukhera Sheikh, Inithan Ganesaratnam, and Haider Jan, "The Birth of Forceps," *JRSM Short Reports* 4, no. 7 (July 2013): 1–4, https://www.ncbi.nlm.nih.gov/pmc/articles/PMC3704058.

and Greek mythology to Hindu, Egyptian, and European folklore. Contrary to popular belief, Julius Caesar was not born by this method. The name comes from an edict during Roman times that a baby should be cut out of a dead or dying woman's body in an attempt to save the baby's life. It was not often successful.[15] By the mid-twentieth century, caesarean section became a more favoured mode of delivery when labour was not progressing and largely replaced forceps deliveries, especially when the baby was not well down in the birth canal.

Modern medicine brought about other changes. Childbirth became a medical procedure, designed to improve outcomes: healthier babies, mothers who survived childbirth. As medicalization took hold, a common sentiment was that "a delivery is normal only in retrospect." Natural childbirth was deemed primitive and unsafe.

Of course, medical procedures themselves have risks. Caesarean section carries the risks of any surgical procedure. Poorly applied forceps can cause injury to the baby, from bruises to nerve damage, and lacerations to the mother. The routine episiotomy was introduced as a way of controlling the tearing of the perineal structure and to give more room for the application of forceps. But as mentioned earlier, the idea that episiotomy heals better than a tear has been shown to be false in well-controlled studies. There is no clear evidence that routine episiotomy provides any benefit to the baby or the mother.[16]

Routine electronic fetal monitoring actually increases risk by dramatically increasing C-section rates and other interventions.[17,]

15   U.S. National Library of Medicine, "Cesarean Section—A Brief History: Part I," History of Medicine, last modified July 26, 2013, https://www.nlm.nih.gov/exhibition/cesarean/part1.html.

16   Hong Jiang, Xu Qian, Guillermo Carroli, and Paul Garner, "Selective versus Routine Use of Episiotomy for Vaginal Birth," *Cochrane Database of Systematic Reviews* 2, no. 2 (February 8, 2017): CD000081, https://www.cochrane.org/CD000081/PREG_selective-versus-routine-use-episiotomy-vaginal-birth.

17   Rebecca Dekker and Anna Bertone, "The Evidence on: Fetal Monitoring," Evidence Based Birth, last modified May 21, 2018, https://evidencebasedbirth.com/fetal-monitoring/, and Ruth Martis, Ova Emilia, Detty S. Nurdiati, and Julie Brown, "Intermittent Auscultation (IA) of Fetal Heart Rate in Labour for Fetal Well-Being," Cochrane Database of Systematic Reviews 2, no. 2 (February 13, 2017): CD008680, https://www.cochranelibrary.com/cdsr/doi/10.1002/14651858.CD008680.pub2/abstract.

Infection control was one of the most significant advances in obstetrical care. Long before germs were discovered, Dr. Ignaz Semmelweis noted that when doctors in his hospital delivered the babies, mothers had much higher rates of the often fatal childbed fever than when midwives performed the deliveries. The Vienna Maternity Hospital where he worked had two wings, one run by doctors and medical students, and the other by midwives. In 1847, in what amounted to a randomized trial, women were admitted on alternate days to either wing. In addition to delivering the babies, the medical students also did postmortem examinations of the women who had died of childbed fever—without changing clothes or washing their hands. Semmelweis surmised that there was something the students were doing that was spreading illness to the women in labour and suggested the students wash their hands in a caustic solution. When the students washed their hands, the instance of childbed fever was reduced by 90 percent. Nevertheless, the idea of stopping to wash their hands was deemed a ludicrous waste of time by the doctors. Gentlemen were not dirty. Semmelweis was ridiculed and condemned.[18]

Joseph Lister, by 1890, had brought the ideas of sterilizing equipment, cleaning hands, and using sterile techniques to popularity, and those ideas spread to obstetrical care. Full surgical sterile field became standard. Draping, gloves, gown and mask, and tying down the mother's hands so she could not contaminate the field of the delivery became the norm in the delivery room.[19] There continued to be advances in obstetrical care. Neonatal management and resuscitation improved survival and decreased morbidity. But the fact remained that a lot of procedures were done simply "because

---

18   Rebecca Davis, "The Doctor Who Championed Hand-Washing and Briefly Saved Lives," NPR, January 12, 2015, https://www.npr.org/sections/health-shots/2015/01/12/375663920/the-doctor-who-championed-hand-washing-and-saved-women-s-lives.

19   Graeme E. Glass, "Beyond Antisepsis: Examining the Relevance of the Works of Joseph Baron Lister to the Contemporary Surgeon-Scientist," *Indian Journal of Plastic Surgery* 47, no. 3 (Sep–Dec 2014): 407–411, https://www.ncbi.nlm.nih.gov/pmc/articles/PMC4292121.

we have always done them." This was particularly true in North America, where the medicalization of birthing was almost universal. In much of Europe and around the world, most normal deliveries were still done by midwives, with less intervention.

Medical care has always had the goal of reducing suffering, and seeing the pain women suffered during labour inspired doctors to find ways to alleviate it. As techniques and medications for anaesthesia in surgery became available, they found their way into labour and delivery.

In 1853, Queen Victoria was administered chloroform for the birth of Prince Leopold, and as a result, the use of anaesthetic for childbirth became popular. It was dubbed "chloroform a la reine."[20] Other pain control medications were developed, as well. Twilight sleep, first described in 1902, was a concoction of two medications (scopolamine and morphine) which gave the woman complete amnesia of the event of the birth. She just came to the hospital and went home with a week-old baby. Suffragettes advocated for a woman's right to have twilight sleep for her delivery.[21]

Spinals and then epidurals gained popularity in obstetrical care in the 1970s, allowing the mother to be awake but without pain—and without the ability to participate in the birth, so forceps and episiotomies became standard. All of these advancements were welcome, but not without problems themselves. Twilight sleep could cause long-term drowsiness and disorientation. Spinal anaesthetic could cause terrible headaches and sometimes nerve damage. Epidurals required another layer of monitoring and could lengthen the total time for labour. Narcotics cross the placenta and could cause breathing problems for the baby, increasing the need for resuscitation.

---

20   Ann Whitfield, "A Short History of Obstetric Anaesthesia," *Res Medica Journal of the Royal Medical Society* 3, no. 1 (1992): 28–30, http://journals.ed.ac.uk/resmedica/article/download/972/1399.

21   Lauren MacIvor Thompson, "The Politics of Female Pain: Women's Citizenship, Twilight Sleep and the Early Birth Control Movement," *Medical Humanities* 45, no. 1 (March 2019): 67–74, https://pubmed.ncbi.nlm.nih.gov/30266831/.

In his book *Childbirth Without Fear*,[22] written in the 1940s, British obstetrician Grantly Dick-Read wrote about the horror of routine anaesthetic + episiotomy + forceps delivery as practiced in North America. Dr. Dick-Read wrote that childbirth was a natural physiological process not meant to be painful. He discussed the effect fear has on the body, increasing muscle tension and decreasing circulation, and the detrimental consequences in childbirth. He described beautifully the natural emotional stages of labour: elation early on; relaxation of the body during active labour; total concentration during the second, or pushing stage; and exaltation at the third stage, right after the baby is born. He explained how these emotional stages are masked by modern practice. By providing education, relaxation, and emotional support for the pregnant woman, he showed that fear could be reduced, the need for anaesthetic decreased, and satisfaction in childbirth increased.

In 1951 Dr. Fernand Lamaze brought the concept of psychoprophylaxis from Russia to France, a method of preparing women for childbirth without anaesthetic by means of education, psychological and physical conditioning, and breathing exercises. Dr. Pierre Vellay, a protege of Dr. Lamaze, wrote *Childbirth Without Pain* in 1960.[23] Marjorie Karmel wrote *Thank You Dr. Lamaze: A Mother's Experience in Painless Childbirth* in 1965,[24] popularizing the Lamaze technique of preparing for childbirth among the North American public.

By taking advantage of all of the advances in medical science, but introducing the ideas Lamaze and others promoted, women were reclaiming control of their experiences around birth. The principles of autonomy, educated choice for women, and inclusion of the husband and family or other loved ones in the birthing led to the concept of family-centred maternity care.

---

22   Grantly Dick-Read, *Childbirth without Fear: The Original Approach to Natural Childbirth* (London: Heinemann Medical Books, 1942).

23   Pierre Vellay, *Childbirth without Pain* (New York: E. P. Dutton & Co., 1960).

24   Marjorie Karmel, *Thank You Dr. Lamaze: A Mother's Experience in Painless Childbirth* (New York: Doubleday, 1965).

Generations of women were not actively involved in the births of their babies. They were anaesthetized, and the medical system took control. That meant there were no role models, no support for the next generation of mothers. The new techniques of preparing for childbirth were actually a way of returning to some of the traditional supports and inherent female knowledge, even while medical advances improved outcomes.

Sheila Kitzinger was a well-known British natural childbirth activist and writer of over twenty books about childbirth. She popularized the relaxation and breathing exercises promoted by Dr. Lamaze. She wrote, "For far too many, pregnancy and birth is still something that happens to them rather than something they set out consciously and joyfully to do themselves."[25]

Kitzinger also wrote:

> Birth, like death, is an experience in which we all share. It can either be a disruption in the flow of human existence, a fragment which has little or nothing to do with loving and being loved or with the passionate longing which created the baby, or it can be lived with beauty and dignity, and labour itself be a celebration of joy. Birth is a part of a woman's very wide psychosexual experiences and is intimately concerned with her feelings about and sense of her own body, her relations with others, her role as a woman, and the meaning of her personal identity. I feel that in choosing to write about childbirth I am at the hub of life.[26]

There were a few doctors who were on board with all of this. Elisabeth Bing, a childbirth education pioneer in the 1960s who cofounded Lamaze International, was quoted in the *Journal of Perinatal Education*:

---

25   Sheila Kitzinger, *The Experience of Childbirth* (New York: Penguin, 1984), 9.

26   Encyclopedia.com, s.v. "Kitzinger, Sheila 1929–," accessed March 27, 2022, https://www.encyclopedia.com/arts/educational-magazines/kitzinger-sheila-1929.

These doctors were prepared to stick their necks out even though there was a lot of opposition from their colleagues at that time to "this crazy fad" and probably because of the climate of the times as well. I think they were uneasy about the overmedication of women and they probably had the same feeling that we had—that there must be better ways. One also has to understand that it was probably the times as well. It was a time when there were many changes going on—women's lib, the Vietnam war, the "flower children," the freedom rides, etc. People seemed to say, "We have to change things; things are not good enough." Prepared childbirth was easy to introduce in a way because the atmosphere was right.[27]

We have embraced the concept of evidence-based medicine and best practices in obstetrics. This has many benefits but also a downside: if something has not been studied in the prescribed way, it's not a "best practice" any longer, and some of the important knowledge and traditional healing ways are marginalized.

Midwives are common around the world and continue to be the birth attendants in many places. In North America, they were diminished and marginalized for a long time. They were common in Indigenous, Mennonite, and other communities but not part of mainstream medical practice.

Again, my father had some influence here. After being asked to testify about a case involving a legal issue around midwifery, he took on the cause and, with others, helped to form a licencing body and college with standards for midwifery in Canada. Up until that point, the use of midwives had become "alegal": not illegal, but also not recognized as part of provincial health care and therefore not funded. Women wanting to use a midwife had to pay out of pocket. In 1994, Ontario and Alberta became the first provinces to regulate and licence midwives. Midwifery is now licenced across

---

27   Elaine Zwelling, "The History of Lamaze Continues: An Interview with Elisabeth Bing," *The Journal of Perinatal Education* 9, no. 1 (Winter 2000): 15–21, https://www.ncbi.nlm.nih.gov/pmc/articles/PMC1595002/.

most of Canada and fully funded through the universal healthcare system. Today, midwives in Canada are required to have professional training and use the same standards of practice that physicians do, the biggest difference being a more patient-focused, one-on-one approach. Midwives are more likely to be involved in home deliveries, but many deliver in hospital settings.

The pendulum swings. Things that were "normal" become "extreme" or "weird" and back again. Caesarean section rates are on the upswing, sometimes even a matter of patient choice. The use of epidural anaesthetic is higher now than it was twenty years ago. What is "normal" is always in flux in the care of the pregnant woman and the delivery of her baby.

Palliative Care

At the other end of life, the pendulum swings as well. What is considered "normal" changes with the times. In the old days, death was seen as a part of life. If a person was lucky enough to avoid the accidents that most succumbed to, at the end of his life, he would take to his bed; family would come and get the old person's words of wisdom and his blessing. The family, usually the women, would provide care, and pain was a part of the reality. A doctor had little to offer for pain, other than laudanum (a precursor of morphine), a gentle word, and a hand to hold.

Infections and trauma were the usual causes of death—along with childbirth. Cancer existed as well, but most people died before it could take hold. The average life expectancy in 1900 was forty-seven years.[28] The only way to treat traumatic injury was to wait and let the body heal or to remove the affected limb. The introduction of antibiotics changed all of that. Wounds were treated with sulfa

---

28   Aaron O'Neill, "Life Expectancy (from Birth) in Canada, from 1800 to 2020," *Statista*, September 6, 2019, https://www.statista.com/statistics/1041135/life-expectancy-canada-all-time/.

starting in 1935[29] and penicillin in 1942,[30] and advances in surgery and anaesthetic changed the treatment and outcome of injuries. War always has a way of advancing medical care, it seems. Nursing care, antibiotics, and treatment for lung damage (caused by mustard gas in World War I) were all discovered due to the afflictions of war. We are quite a species, aren't we?

By 1950, the life expectancy in North America was 68 years, and by 2000, it was 76.7 years.[31] Probably the greatest impact on our increase in life expectancy has been in the public health realm: immunization, clean water, better hygiene, better nutrition. Changes in our Western diet, technology, and modern work-saving conveniences came at a price, though, and now cardiovascular diseases are the number one killers in our society. With the longevity and environmental changes progress has offered us, cancer kills many more people now than it did a century ago.

There was a shift, not only in life expectancy but in where people died. In 1900, the vast majority of deaths occurred in the home in North America. By 1950, 50 percent of deaths occurred in institutions. And by 1980, only 25 percent of deaths occurred at home. A survey in 2018 showed 60 percent of Canadians die in hospitals, although only 15 percent said they would choose to do so.[32] We have developed ways of treating cancer, with radiation and chemotherapy and advanced surgical techniques. We have also developed advances in cardiac care, from basic CPR to advanced cardiac life support, anticoagulation agents, and treatment of hypertension and diabetes. Intensive care units have evolved as more and more high-level

---

29   "Gerhard Domagk," Science History Institute, last modified December 4, 2017, https://www.sciencehistory.org/historical-profile/gerhard-domagk.

30   Robert Gaynes, "The Discovery of Penicillin—New Insights After More Than 75 Years of Clinical Use," Emerging Infectious Diseases 23, no. 5 (May 2017): 849–853, https://www.ncbi.nlm.nih.gov/pmc/articles/PMC5403050/.

31   "North American Life Expectancy 1950–2022," Macrotrends, accessed March 27, 2022, https://www.macrotrends.net/countries/NAC/north-america/life-expectancy.

32   Celina Carter, "What It's Really Like to Die at Home in Ontario," Healthy Debate, June 27, 2019, https://healthydebate.ca/2019/06/topic/dying-at-home/.

treatments have emerged. We have machines that measure heart rate, respiration, and oxygen levels, and we have monitors for blood pressure, fluid balances, brain activity, renal activity, and on and on. Specialized nursing and specialized medical care require intensive observation and treatment, and it has become more efficient to have the equipment and the expertise in special rooms in hospitals.

Visitors and family are relegated to waiting rooms and allowed in to see their loved ones only for short periods of time, so as not to interfere with the lifesaving treatments going on in the ICU.

With the medicalization of birth, deliveries became "normal only in retrospect." Similarly, there was a shift in attitudes toward death. The acceptance that dying was a normal event, a part of every family's story, gave way to the notion that every death was a failure of medicine. As more deaths occurred away from home, personal exposure to death and dying decreased. It is now a distant, unknown, and feared event. In our time, most people have never seen a dead person.

Once it became obvious that the battle to cure an individual's cancer or other illness was lost, the medical system gave up on that person. "There is nothing more we can do" became the pronouncement, and the person was relegated to a back hall and basically just left to die. Pain was poorly treated; there was no priority given to the spiritual or mental well-being of the person. Or, as I described earlier, patients were shifted to the ICU so medical teams could pull out all the stops and keep the person alive at all costs. Death was the enemy, and every death was a failure.

More and more people were dying in ICUs, surrounded by strangers, flashing lights, and tubes out of every orifice, and ending their lives with a failed cardiac resuscitation attempt. There arose a new pushback, a new advocacy to take back the human aspect of dying. Just as with the natural childbirth movement, many people began to demand some choice, some autonomy, and some dignity in the dying process. The AIDS epidemic of the 1980s brought about some advocacy for the care of the dying, but this was largely a fringe movement.

In her book *On Death and Dying*, in 1969, Elisabeth Kübler-Ross[33] wrote about the psychological stages a dying person goes through. Around the same time in Britain, Dame Cicely Saunders was horrified by how poorly the dying patients were being treated in her hospital. As a nurse, she felt so helpless that she went back to school and became a social worker, then a physician, and dedicated her life to the care of the dying. In 1967, she founded St. Christopher's Hospice in London, England. Dame Cicely said, "You matter because you are you, and you matter to the end of your life. We will do all we can not only to help you die peacefully, but also to live until you die."[34] This promise became the basic tenet of palliative care.

The term "hospice" dates back to the Crusades, "when monasteries provided refuge not only for the sick and dying, but for weary travellers, labouring women, the poor, orphans, and lepers."[35] Dr. Saunders described modern hospice as care centred on the person, their whole health—mental, physical, spiritual, relational—while promoting the use of narcotics for pain control in cancer.

Dr. Balfour Mount first brought the focus on care for the dying patient to North America after visiting St. Christopher's Hospice. He coined the term palliative care in the 1970s, feeling that the term hospice carried the stigma of a last resort for the poor and derelict. He opened the first palliative care unit in North America in the Royal Victoria Hospital in Montreal, Quebec. Around the same time, a similar unit opened at St. Boniface Hospital in Winnipeg, Manitoba.[36]

---

33   Elisabeth Kübler-Ross, *On Death and Dying: What the Dying Have to Teach Doctors, Nurses, Clergy and Their Own Families* (New York: Scribner, 1969).

34   "Annual Report 2016," Hospice and Palliative Care Services, accessed March 27, 2022, https://www.hospicare.org/wp-content/uploads/2017/07/2016-AR-POSTCARD-PP2.pdf.

35   Katherine Arnup, "Contemporary Family Trends: Death, Dying and Canadian Families," The Vanier Institute of the Family, 2013, https://vanierinstitute.ca/wp-content/uploads/2015/12/CFT_2013-11-00_EN.pdf.

36   "History," Palliative Care McGill, accessed March 27, 2022, https://www.mcgill.ca/palliativecare/about-us/history.

According to the World Health Organization (WHO), palliative care is the approach to care meant to improve quality of life for patients and their families when faced with life-threatening illness. It involves the relief of suffering and the treatment of pain, whether physical, psychosocial, or spiritual. Palliative caregivers focus upon a patient-centred team approach in providing care and support, from practical needs to bereavement counselling, encouraging the principle of living as actively as possible until death. Palliative care is explicitly recognized under the human right to health. Its focus is on comfort rather than cure.[37]

To some, hospice is the physical building where care can be provided away from the hospital as an alternative to home itself, equivalent to a birthing centre for low-risk obstetrical care. Some jurisdictions define hospice within a specific time frame prior to death or once treatment is no longer an option, while palliative care is a looser concept.

In Canada, the two terms are largely used interchangeably, and the organization promoting this approach is called the Canadian Hospice Palliative Care Association.

It used to be that all family doctors did deliveries. For various reasons, specialists have taken over the majority of obstetrical care. Similarly, until recently, doctors cared for their patients right up until death. But as more and more people were dying in hospitals and in ICUs, this aspect of care moved away from family doctors.

We are still very much a death-denying society; it's uncomfortable to have to deal with these patients and their many needs. I think the battle to have obstetrical care return to the realm of the family doctor is pretty much lost, although I sincerely hope not. Family medicine residency programmes promote low-risk primary care obstetrics again, but numbers continue to decline. Obstetricians now do a majority of the normal low-risk deliveries, midwives are increasingly taking up the slack, and few GPs want the irregular hours, complexity, and messiness of childbirth.

---

37   "Palliative Care," World Health Organization, August 5, 2020, https://www.who.int/news-room/fact-sheets/detail/palliative-care.

The same thing is occurring in the care of the dying. The rise of palliative care as a speciality means that many family doctors feel less capable of caring for their dying patients on their own, especially in the management of complex pain. Teaching the skills needed for this vital aspect of family medicine is key.

Just as in the advocacy surrounding birth, the movement toward palliative care aimed to bring some humanity back to dying, with a return to a more patient-centred, family-centred approach, while not abandoning the many medical advances available to treat disease and save lives. Excellence in pain and symptom control is important. So is allowing people to think, feel, fear, love, communicate. The involvement of family, the concept of personal choice in treatment options, of education, is just like the consumer movement that brought about the family-centred maternity care of the 1960s.

Tokothanatology

The care provided in both maternity and end-of-life settings has swung from one extreme to another and is swinging more to the centre for both. What is "normal" ebbs and flows; what is in fashion will continue to swing one way and then the other. The principles are the same, though. We strive to use the best practices and the best advances in technique while embracing the human experience, the softer side of what a person wants and needs during these journeys.

There is not a formal branch of medicine called tokothanatology (yet). I have met many people who provided care in childbirth and switched to palliative care later in their careers, and many who practice both simultaneously. Doctors, nurses, doulas, social workers, and others have made the connection that is tokothanatology, whether consciously or not. The art of medicine takes on such a vital role at these extremes of life, perhaps more than at any other stage, and the skills of care at one end enhance the practice at the other.

Many world religions weigh in on the continuity of the life cycle, from reincarnation to the concept of the soul entering and leaving human form. And there is a body of literature about ethical questions around life, birth, and death.

I was able to find very little written about this concept from a healthcare perspective. I found just one book: *Birth and Death: Experience, Ethics, Politics,* by sociologists Kath Woodward and Sophie Woodward (2020).[38] They argued that "both are central to our experiences of being in the world and part of living." *Birth to Death: Science and Bioethics* is a collection of essays edited by David Thomasma and Thomasine Kushner.[39] And Sholom Glouberman, Philosopher in Residence at Baycrest Home for the Aged in Toronto and president of the Patients Canada, wrote an essay in the *Journal of Evaluation in Clinical Practice* called "The Grey Zones of Birth and Death" (2011), about the interactions between scientific advances and the human aspects of birth and death.[40] There are likely more that I haven't come across. Through my own book, I hope to spread awareness among the medical and healthcare communities, drawing attention to the similarities between these sentinel events in every person's life.

---

38   Kath Woodward and Sophie Woodward, *Birth and Death: Experience, Ethics, Politics* (New York: Routledge, 2020).

39   David C. Thomasma and Thomasine Kushner. eds., *Birth to Death, Science and Bioethics* (Cambridge: Cambridge University Press, 1996).

40   Sholom Glouberman, "The Grey Zones of Birth and Death," *Journal of Evaluation in Clinical Practice* 17, no. 2 (April 2011): 394–399, https://www.researchgate.net/journal/Journal-of-Evaluation-in-Clinical-Practice-1365-2753.

CHAPTER 3

Principles of Family-Centred Maternity Care and of Palliative Care

The good physician treats the disease;
the great physician treats the patient who has the disease.
—William Osler

Tokothanatology: Consumer movements have shaped the care we provide for women giving birth by increasing patient involvement in decision-making and drawing the whole family into the circle of care. Palliative care similarly seeks to involve patients, along with their families, to allow more personal control in decisions as they deal with their last days.

VALMAI ELKINS WROTE *THE RIGHTS OF THE PREGNANT PARENT* IN 1976 as a call to arms for pregnant couples to take back control of their childbirth experience.[41] I've taken the liberty of summarizing her ideas.

41   Valmai Elkins, *The Rights of the Pregnant Parent* (New York: Schocken Press, 1976).

The Pregnant Parent's Bill of Rights

You have the right to a safe delivery of your child.

You have the right to receive the best evidence-based medical care for you and your baby.

You have the right to knowledge about your pregnancy and delivery and the options for delivery.

You have the right to choose who will deliver your baby.

You have the right to include the support people of your choice at the birth.

You have the right to choose the location of the birth.

You have the right to use the pain control techniques of your choice during labour.

You have the right to decide about medication or epidural when available and to be informed of the risks and benefits of these interventions.

You have the right to refuse treatments and the right to be informed of the risks of any refusal to you and to your baby.

You have the right to deliver in a position of your choosing.

You have the right of access to your baby at all times.

You have the right to be informed of any procedures done to your baby and the reasons for them.

You have the right to receive support in feeding your baby in the way you choose.

You have the right to follow-up care for you and for your baby in the postpartum period and beyond.

Elkins encouraged couples to write out birth plans to discuss with their doctor. The plans would outline the things couples felt were most important to them based on the rights Elkins talked about in her book. *Who would a woman have with her during labour? What medications would she like to use for pain? Would she like to squat for pushing?* and so on. These kinds of questions were meant to open up conversations with the doctor; however, at the time, some women presented their birth plans as a list of demands, and some doctors took the plans as an affront to their expertise. Many things could change expectations during labour. Some wishes might not be feasible in a particular situation. A woman's stamina or her pain tolerance may not be what she had anticipated. Sometimes hospital policies didn't allow certain practices, and sometimes the doctor's level of comfort was pushed too far.

Eventually, the idea of a birth plan evolved into a way of sharing information between patient and caregiver, with the understanding that it is not possible to know how a particular labour will unfold. Part of the conversation should be about dealing with this uncertainty and building trust that the patient's wishes are heard and acknowledged. Many of the things women in the 1960s had to fight for are now the normal practice.

Similarly, when a person is facing a terminal illness, dying has become medicalized; the doctors have become the decision-makers. Patients and their families need to feel they are a part of the process. To help start a discussion, a bill of rights for the palliative patient could look like this:

The Dying Person's Bill of Rights

You have the right to the best medical care available during your illness.

You have the right to access to information about your illness, treatment choices, and potential benefits and risks, as well as side effects of any treatment choices.

You have the right to an open discussion about alternative treatments.

You have the right to ongoing care by modern medicine while also engaging in alternative treatments if you so choose.

You have the right to refuse any intervention and the right to know the likely outcome with and without treatment, and how either approach could affect your comfort and quality of life.

You have the right to be informed of any test results.

You have the right to adequate pain and symptom control.

You have the right to include the support people of your choice.

You have the right to be cared for in the place of your choice.

You have the right to emotional support for yourself and your family and loved ones.

You have the right to access to spiritual support.

You have the right to access to legal support concerning financial matters and end-of-life care.

You have the right to receive support for your family and loved ones in their bereavement after your death.

As you can see, the rights and wishes of people who are facing the end of their lives mirror a lot of those of childbearing women. Once again, these "rights" are meant to be a way to open up discussion with the doctor, not a list of demands. Remember that sometimes hospital policies are in disagreement, or sometimes the doctor's comfort level is challenged, but discussion around this bill of rights could be a way of coming to a mutual understanding. Births and deaths are going to take place regardless of any intervention. The goal then is not to change the outcome—the birth of this child, the death of this individual—but rather to make the experience the best it can be. There are certain common threads that help. The role of the medical practitioner has evolved from the paternalistic, one-and-only decision maker to a partner in the decision-making process, an educator and support person.

Sharing information with the patient is essential. The "doctor knows best" attitude has little place in healthcare any longer. But we do have the education and the knowledge, and it is vital that we share our expertise, to give the patient and her family the information they need. Doing so takes time, and because these are emotionally overwhelming periods in a person's life, information needs to be repeated and reinforced.

Even the most highly educated person goes numb when faced with a drastic change in their life, whether it is the start of a new family or the loss of a life. I often found it helpful to write some notes for the person to take away, and I reinforced the offer to go over things again, to give ample time for questions, and even to suggest what questions patients might want to ask.

"What happens now? What options do I have? Is it worthwhile getting a second opinion? Is there something I can read about this?" To involve the patient in the decision-making process means they must have enough information to be able to know what to ask. Education helps, on what is expected at each stage of a pregnancy or an illness and what the likely outcomes of any intervention will be, both positive and negative. It should also touch on hospital policies, medications, investigations, treatment, and options about where care can be given.

During childbirth, things can change very quickly, and intervention can make a huge difference in the safety of mother or baby. In palliative care, discussion before any crisis situation is also useful so that the person's wishes for intervention are known and documented. I can't tell you how many times I was called on to make decisions about a medical crisis in the middle of the night. As a doctor on call, I may not know the patient or her wishes, so I would be obligated to start resuscitation efforts which might very well be contrary to the patient's goals. Communication with other members of the extended care team and with family is vital so that everyone is on the same page at any time. Much like a birth plan, advance directives, living wills, and powers of attorney are tools for discussing a person's wishes in advance.

It happens less commonly than in the past, but sometimes family members wish to hide from a person the fact that they are dying, fearing they will give up hope. In reality, most patients know what is happening to them and welcome the chance to face the fact out loud and with supportive people. Those who do not may keep their thoughts to themselves, to protect their family and ensure loved ones will not give up on them.

I called this the conspiracy of silence. My father described it so very well about his parents. He was a medical student when his mother lay dying of cancer. Both parents insisted that he not tell the other. "It would kill him," his mother said. "It would kill her," said his father. Three quarters of a century later, my father still recalled that time with pain.

Truth-telling is an ethical issue. Telling enough so the person understands and can accommodate the information, and in a kind rather than abrupt manner, takes some balancing. It may take a few conversations. It is common to be asked for the same information on numerous occasions. And some people never hear, or never want to know.

Different family members may be at different stages of acceptance. Often one family member, sometimes the one with unresolved conflict, is not willing or able to "give up" and allow treatment to be stopped. Family meetings, having everybody together to hear and discuss plans, are useful here.

In maternity care, as well, promoting open communication between the parents about their emotions, fears, and hopes encourages them to support each other and reveal hidden conflicts. Taking time during prenatal visits to delve into some of these things can pay dividends.

Helping children understand what is happening, whether about their mother's pregnancy or when a loved one is ill, is something a family doctor can facilitate. Discussions about a family member's terminal illness should be age-specific and as open as possible, recognizing the impact such an event can have on children's' lives. Siblings should be part of the pregnancy conversation, especially when there are difficulties with the pregnancy or the baby. Children are sometimes forgotten in the turmoil, their emotional needs and understanding of the situation neglected.

Inherent in the principles of patient-centred care at both ends of life is the awareness and respect for personal preferences, cultural practices, and treatment choices. I always encouraged my patients to tell me anything they were doing outside of my suggestions, and noted it in a nonjudgemental way. Honest discussion about these practices and requests is so important.

Pioneers of the childbirth education movement stressed the interaction of fear and pain in labour. Knowledge about the progress of normal labour is a key to decreasing fear, and thus decreasing pain. The influence of emotions is worth exploring in end-of-life care as well. If left unaddressed, they can affect decision-making, exacerbate pain, and get in the way of communication. Pain is worsened when existential suffering is not addressed. And existential suffering is worsened when pain is not addressed.

Living through the final stages of a loved one's life will have a profound effect on survivors' grieving and their future lives. Similarly, stories or experiences of labour and delivery can have an effect on parenting and future birth experiences.

In order to remain objective, doctors often feel the need to be detached and clinical. But dealing with a person on a human level means making a commitment to the person as a whole being—not just a uterus, not just a disease. Part of our job is to care. Yet, while being involved, we must also maintain our objectivity so that we can be effective and not detract from our patient's journey. It is a delicate balancing act. Even the best doctors can get the balance wrong occasionally.

Guilty as charged. I sometimes found myself overwhelmed by my patient's story to the detriment of my own clarity. Fortunately, I had a very astute and supportive husband who would call me on it and remind me to maintain some objectivity. He also pointed out that I was the most emotionally overwrought when death and pregnancy intertwined, and of course he was always right.

Support for the family is inherent in the principles of family-centred maternity care and in palliative care. Equally important, the family is part of the care team. The patient is integrated with other people and their opinions and needs. Relationships have an impact on how people cope with symptoms, how they relate to professionals, and how and why they make decisions. The person at the centre of this—the one giving birth, the one at the end of life—should have some control over who is in her circle of care.

The definition of family goes beyond the traditional here, to include any of the people with whom the patient feels a strong relationship. It could mean nontraditional partners, relatives, friends, coworkers, or neighbours.

Imagine delivering a baby and then just leaving the mother and baby to fend for themselves. It sounds ridiculous and uncaring. A care team's involvement with the family does not end with the delivery of the baby and does not end at the deathbed. The concept of family-centred care includes support and care leading up to and after the events at both ends of life. One of the rights of the dying is to know that his loved ones will be supported after his death. The moment of death, just like the moment of birth, is only part of the continuum, and care should envelop the time before, during, and afterward.

By definition, the family dynamic always shifts at the beginning and ending of a life.

With a new baby, couples become parents. Children become siblings with new places in the family structure. Parents become grandparents.

When a person receives the diagnosis of a terminal illness, their family likewise makes a major shift in its dynamics. Primary wage earners might become dependants. Adult children become parent figures. Fathers might have to take over childcare and household roles. When a child is severely ill, the other children may find their own issues put on hold. And a spousal role can change from equal partner to caregiver. Family relationships may take on deeper meaning; this can be a time for resolving conflicts, if handled correctly. Often, simply a gentle suggestion on the part of a professional can open the door to a meaningful conversation that can be so valuable for the survivor's emotional well-being later in life. Sometimes the family doctor can have a role in facilitating these conversations. Sometimes a social worker, a spiritual support person, or a counsellor can be brought in.

Some families will be actively involved in the physical care of the dying person. Their own needs must be met, and their wishes are as significant as the patient's. If a person wishes to die at home, the family has to be on board, willing and able to do the lion's share of the actual care.

A conflict I saw over and over had to do with accepting further, often futile treatment. For example, a husband may feel he wants to give in and accept the reality of his dying, but his wife clings to the possibility that chemotherapy might keep him alive. In some cases, he might go ahead with treatment just to please her.

A patient's adult children may have very different opinions about treatment, too. Sometimes, a child with unresolved issues with an ill parent is the one who fights hardest to keep the parent alive, in an attempt to smooth over past differences or to alleviate their own mixed or painful feelings. Again, family meetings may help address these conflicts, along with input from others in the circle.

Care teams include many different medical professionals along with nonmedical support people and family members. Childbirth educators, nurses, and doulas work alongside the doctor or midwife throughout pregnancy, labour and delivery, and into newborn care and breastfeeding support. At the end of life, nurses and doctors, chaplains, spiritual advisors, social workers, and lawyers are added into the team structure. Palliative care volunteers and death doulas, also called end-of-life or EOL doulas, often have a role to play in supporting the dying person and his family.

Birth doula care is described as a relationship with the expectant family, giving encouragement, supporting the client's wishes during the whole process of giving birth, and providing the key component of continuous attendance. In death and dying, doula care can provide this same continuous level of advocacy and support, helping with planning, communicating with the medical team, and improving satisfaction. Research has shown that, both in birth and death, a nonmedical emotional support person improves outcomes and provides higher levels of satisfaction, lower costs, and less uncertainty with interventions.[42]

As you can see, many of these principles share common threads in the care we give at the two extremes of life. While it is not in our power to change the fact that these events will happen, we can have a positive influence on the transitions for patients and their families, providing education, support, guidance, and empathy. Understanding some of the softer sides of birth and death will serve to enhance this impact.

---

42   Francesca Arnoldy, "The End-of-Life Doula Movement," *Today's Geriatric Medicine* 12, no. 1 (January/February 2019): 12, https://www.todaysgeriatricmedicine.com/archive/JF19p12.shtml.

CHAPTER 4

Psychological, Spiritual, and Socioeconomic Aspects of Childbirth and Death

You don't have a soul. You are a soul. You have a body.
—C.S. Lewis

Tokothanatology: Birth and death are defining events in people's lives. While the birth of a child generally brings optimism and happiness to a family, and the death of a loved one may bring sadness and emptiness, these events have many complex emotions in common. As well, there are many social and economic changes that impact families when a birth or a death occurs.

MY MOTHER OFTEN TOLD A STORY ABOUT HER SECOND pregnancy. She described the overwhelming feeling of love she had felt for her firstborn (me) as soon as the baby was born and how the love grew as time went on. Pregnant with her second child, she felt a bit of sadness for this new baby growing within her, as she thought she could not possibly feel the same strong love she felt for me. But as soon as my sister arrived, my mother realized that the love increased exponentially, and she had just as much love for her second baby as she had for her first. A sense of relief along with the love made the emotional connection even stronger. My mother said this surge of love repeated itself with each of her babies, and I know she felt it completely for all four of us for her whole life.

Along with the physical changes a person undergoes, many other factors influence childbirth and dying. The people in their lives, the amount of money they have, their race or ethnicity, and their education are all important. A lot of work has been done to improve safety and physical comfort at both ends of life. But we also need to understand how the outside world and the psychological makeup of a person shapes the care they receive.

Obstetrical care focuses on tools to improve the outcomes of a healthy mother and baby, along with a pain-free and safe delivery. Awareness of the emotional aspects of pregnancy and childbirth is also vital. As a caregiver, discussing life's stresses and emotions during pregnancy and offering support can be helpful. Just asking about and allowing time to share these feelings provides validation.

Bringing a new life into the world is generally a joyful event, greatly anticipated and celebrated, and for many women, an empowering journey of discovery. Planning, anticipating the new addition to the family, and daydreaming about who this child will become are part of the reality of many pregnant parents, along with the designing and planning of a nursery, buying diapers, and choosing a name.

But fears and other negative emotions arise as well. Not all pregnancies are welcome, blessed events in a woman's life. Financial worries, memories of past birth experiences, and family stories may have an impact. The pregnancy may not have been planned. (According to the *Washington Post*, in 2018, 45 percent of pregnancies in the US were unplanned.[43]) The pregnancy may be a result of sexual assault. Or the woman simply may not want to become a parent.

---

43   Karen Weese, "Almost Half of Pregnancies in the U.S. Are Unplanned. There's a Surprisingly Easy Way to Change That," *The Washington Post*, May 1, 2018, https://www.washingtonpost.com/news/posteverything/wp/2018/05/01/almost-half-of-pregnancies-in-the-u-s-are-unplanned-theres-a-surprisingly-easy-way-to-change-that/.

There may be health implications for the mother, perceived or real. She may have ingested alcohol or drugs and may now have feelings of guilt or fear for the health of her baby. There may be fears of miscarriage, or of the changes in body image, or the effect of this baby on the relationship with her partner or with others. Her career plans may be put on hold. These worries can be addressed in the context of a prenatal visit, or occasionally by bringing in more expert help. Listening is acknowledging.

Fear has been shown to increase pain in labour. The principles of family-centred maternity care are based on education and empowerment of the pregnant woman and those around her. Understanding what is happening reduces fear and allows for informed choice about all aspects of pregnancy, labour, delivery, and the newborn baby.

Expectant parents benefit from education about their new role. The reality of parenting is more physically demanding than many realize; the inability to do it all can be overwhelming. There are many excellent parenting books and groups available, and discussing these challenges and options should be part of prenatal visits. Friends and family are the most influential resources, of course—although perhaps less so than in days gone by, because of our more connected, mobile society.

With a terminal illness, education around what to expect is equally important. Knowledge about the disease process, the planned treatments, and ideas for symptom control are vital to the patient and his family.

Body image can cause unhappiness or anxiety for a pregnant woman as her shape changes and she loses her familiar figure. Similarly, a dying person may see his body mass decreasing, his loss of muscle tone a stark reminder of his illness. The psychological aspects of these body changes can affect the person's self-esteem and their relationships with others.

There are many tales of emotional outbursts that husbands endure but don't understand. Pregnancy brain, baby brain, and mommy brain are all terms used to describe the fogginess that many pregnant women and new mothers experience. This condition has been attributed to hormones, although lack of sleep is certainly also a factor.

Fifty to seventy-five percent of women describe some sadness or "baby blues" after their babies are born. Approximately 10–15 percent of women will experience a more severe and long-lasting depression, while about one in one thousand will suffer a postpartum psychosis, with delusions, rapid mood swings, or hallucinations.[44] Most women who suffer from postpartum depression do not harm themselves or their child, but there are tragic stories of women committing suicide or harming their infants, so urgent treatment is crucial and can be lifesaving. A previous psychotic episode or family history of bipolar disorder may increase the risk of psychosis, so prenatal screening and education is vital.

The psychological effects around death and dying also have a huge impact on the people involved. Dealing with the prospect of dying is an emotional time for a person. So is the prospect of losing a loved one. The full gamut of feelings comes into play for all involved, just as it does with the birth of a child.

Recall that in Elisabeth Kübler-Ross's groundbreaking book *On Death and Dying*, she said that denial, anger, bargaining, depression, and acceptance are the emotional stages a dying person goes through.[45] Although she first proposed that there was a progression from one stage to the next, we now understand that these stages occur in no particular order and may change rapidly, or one feeling may last for the rest of a person's life. We are quick to label "where the patient is." Labels can be helpful to a certain extent in understanding how to support the patient or to help the family cope, but they can also be limiting. Much more useful is to listen to what he is saying and deal with that.

---

44   "Postpartum Depression," Cleveland Clinic, last modified January 1, 2018, https://my.clevelandclinic.org/health/diseases/9312-postpartum-depression.

45   Elisabeth Kübler-Ross, *On Death and Dying: What the Dying Have to Teach Doctors, Nurses, Clergy and Their Own Families* (New York: Scribner, 1969), 265.

Initiating palliative care for a patient means acknowledging that a cure is no longer an option. This is a paradigm shift for all involved: the patient, the family, and the professionals. We acknowledge that this disease is likely how the person will die, even as we provide treatment. Dealing with the emotional minefield of fear and anxiety is as important as treating the disease and controlling physical symptoms.

It is not surprising that a person feels distress when facing his own mortality. But not all the emotional changes that occur when a person is dying are negative. Some people feel a sense of peace in allowing themselves to be cared for and in connecting with others on a deeply meaningful level. Some people describe a sense of joy in discovering what is truly important to them, a sweetness in reminiscing about the life they had.

The people surrounding the dying person are impacted on an emotional level, in many ways even more than the patient herself. While the person with the illness only has the inevitable outcome to deal with, the family, friends, coworkers, and caregivers must cope with this dying phase and then with their own lives after the death. Loved ones can go through the same stages that Kübler-Ross describes in the dying patient. Different family members often experience these stages at different times, which can complicate matters further. One family member may be angry, lashing out at others, accusing them of not caring, or not pushing hard enough, or pushing too hard. Another might be sad, but accepting of the situation, and looking toward how to go on after the loved one's death. Healthcare professionals can play an important role in helping families navigate these conflicts.

In much the same way, a woman goes through many different emotions during the course of her pregnancy. Joy, fear, worry, anticipation, love, acceptance, empowerment, and self-doubt are all part of the process. There are many theories about how stress in the pregnant woman affects the developing fetus. High maternal cortisol levels may be linked to preterm birth and an increased incidence of mental health problems in children.[46] But I personally think that emotion-related hormones pass to the fetus in an undifferentiated form and give the baby a sense of involvement with the mother.

Every religion has a story about how life begins and what happens when a person dies. Even the nonreligious have an explanation of life, if only on a molecular level. Rituals are a way of sharing these beliefs, as we will explore in the next chapter.

Finding meaning in the big questions as well as the simple moments that make life, well, alive is what spirituality endeavors to do. How does a collection of cells become a human being? Where does her soul come from? What happens to a person when he dies? Does his soul go to heaven or hell, or is it reincarnated into another life? Is he reunited with ancestors or loved ones, or God, or does he simply stop being? These questions and their answers are the realm of the spiritual. Many religious practices are ways of welcoming a newborn into the community or saying goodbye at the end of a person's life.

To many people, spirituality and religion are one and the same. To others, they are individual concepts. The formal religions in which some people are raised can provide frameworks for their everyday lives and offer answers to the deep questions of life and death. For others, answers to such questions are a lifelong exploration. For still others, the questions only become real when a life is about to end or when a child is born.

A midwife from Nigeria described an interesting cultural spin. In her home country, where infant mortality is high, childbirth is a private, quiet affair, and the baby is openly celebrated only when he begins to crawl. On the other hand, when a person is dying, the whole community celebrates as that individual is "being released" from earthly restraints.[47]

---

46   Elysia Poggi Davis and Curt A. Sandman, "The Timing of Prenatal Exposure to Maternal Cortisol and Psychosocial Stress Is Associated with Human Infant Cognitive Development," *Child Development* 81, no. 1 (January 2010): 131–148, https://www.ncbi.nlm.nih.gov/pmc/articles/PMC2846100/.

47   E. R. Bild, personal communication, 2021.

There is an old saying: "There are no atheists in foxholes." In times of extreme stress such as war, all people will hope for or believe in a higher power.

A number of my dying patients surprised their families by asking for Bible readings, or old hymns, or visits from clergy after years of no involvement in their religious affiliations. We found having a chaplain as part of our palliative care team very useful, as a non-denominational spiritual advisor.

Equally important, though, was the idea that palliative care was not a religious programme. Many patients expressed the fear that "those people will come in and pray over me." They didn't want that, and they were more willing to accept palliative care when assured that no prayer would happen without their explicit request and that no one would try to convert them.

Suffering can have spiritual meaning. Physical pain is easy to see as suffering, but it is shaped by many factors: cultural, emotional, and past experiences. Dame Cicely Saunders talked about total pain as the suffering that encompasses all of a person's physical, psychological, social, spiritual, and practical struggles. Even without physical pain, a person who is facing his demise is likely to experience existential pain or suffering. Eric Cassell discussed this beautifully in his classic book on the subject, *The Nature of Suffering*.[48] He talks about the meaning of pain, not as a strict correlation between the amount of physical pain and the suffering it causes, but taking into account the circumstances and connotations behind the pain. He says the pain of childbirth may be physically severe but means something entirely different than the pain of a tumour pressing on a nerve.

Cassell goes on to say, "A distinction based on clinical observations is made between suffering and physical distress. Suffering is experienced by persons, not merely by bodies." He also wrote, "The perceived meaning of pain influences the amount of medication

48   Eric Cassell, *The Nature of Suffering and the Goals of Medicine* (Oxford: Oxford University Press, 1991).

required to control it. For example, a patient reported that when she believed the pain in her leg was sciatica, she could control it with small doses of codeine, but when she discovered that it was due to the spread of malignant disease, much greater amounts of medication were required for relief."[49]

Some women experience little or no pain during labour. My sister describes feelings of powerful effort, like she would feel on a strenuous hike, during her labour with her second child. She had lower back pain early in labour, but with a gentle touch from the midwife, it disappeared. She remembers an intense burning as she pushed, but nothing she identifies as pain.

There are other well-known examples of this phenomenon. Think of the athlete who runs on a broken ankle and doesn't feel any pain until the end of the race, or the documentation of soldiers who claimed to feel no pain in the heat of battle. Some people experience intractable pain with no evidence of anatomical damage, perhaps attributed to psychological distress and often treated with mental health strategies.

Grantly Dick-Read said, "Many women have described their experiences of childbirth as being associated with a spiritual uplifting, the power of which they have never previously been aware."[50] The overwhelming physical transformation the woman's body undergoes, and the transition from fetus to newborn with all of the physiological changes that must occur, combine with a profound sense of wonder as a new life comes into being. As a doctor, I witnessed it many times, and I never lost my sense of awe at this miracle.

---

49   Eric J. Cassell, "The Nature of Suffering and the Goals of Medicine," *New England Journal of Medicine* 306, no. 11 (March 18, 1982): 369–645, https://www.nejm.org/doi/full/10.1056/NEJM198203183061104.

50   Grantly Dick-Read, *Childbirth without Fear: The Original Approach to Natural Childbirth* (London: Pinter and Martin Ltd., 2004), 25.

EXTERNAL INFLUENCES SUCH AS CULTURE and economic status have a profound effect on the experiences people have at both ends of life.

Poverty, low socioeconomic status, or being a member of a racialized group can contribute to worse outcomes in pregnancy. Decreased access to prenatal care can result in more complications such as lower birth weight and an increase in premature birth and infant or maternal death.

In Canada, parents are guaranteed paid parental leave, which can be taken by either parent, or both, for a total of twelve months.[51] This support does not exist for unemployed or self-employed women at the present time in Canada, but it does in some countries. Estonia mandates eighty-two weeks of paid leave for new parents. Some countries offer maternity leave only, and most of the industrialized world has some sort of paid maternity or parental leave, the notable exception being much of the U.S.[52] Having time to adjust to a new baby without financial concerns can make a huge difference for parents.

While not mandated in Canada, many government programmes and private companies make accommodations for paid leave for caregivers of the terminally ill. These accommodations can ease the financial stress for family caregivers, allowing them to be with their loved ones.

Just as with prenatal care, it is a sad reality that socioeconomic factors affect outcomes of disease, and survival rates are lower in poorer communities. Poverty has an influence on what diseases a person is likely to get, as well. Diabetes, heart disease, and infections are more common and have worse outcomes in the poor than in more privileged members of society. Treatment options, and even vaccinations and other preventive measures, are sadly

---

51 "Employment Insurance Benefits: EI Maternity and Parental Benefits," Government of Canada, last modified April 11, 2022, https://www.canada.ca/en/services/benefits/ei/ei-maternity-parental.html.

52 Marguerite Ward, "10 Countries That Show Just How behind the US Is in Paid Parental Leave for New Mothers and Fathers," *Business Insider*, last modified May 5, 2020, https://www.businessinsider.com/countries-with-best-parental-leave-2016-8.

lacking in many parts of the world. Here in North America, there are gross disparities in health outcomes in Indigenous communities, racialized groups, and Black populations. Public health issues as basic as a lack of clean water and access to care continue to plague portions of Indigenous and remote communities. We as a society have a lot of work to do to improve outcomes in these groups.

Even medical decisions can be shaped by societal expectations. In Brazil, the richest and most highly educated women have the highest rates of elective caesarean section, which gives the impression that C-sections are the best care available. The country's caesarean section rates are among the highest in the world, and C-sections are sought after as the ideal way to give birth.

Similarly, the way people deal with dying is strongly influenced by their background and culture.

Take a look at some examples of cultural influence:

- The Inuit culture is known for having the whole community watching out for and teaching the expectant mother, encouraging her to eat healthy foods and exercise. The baby is very much a community responsibility.

- Indigenous people place a high value on community and relationships, so having contact with the people in their lives becomes very important to the dying. For many, this relationship extends to the land, so being close to their home community takes on meaning for some.

- People of African or Asian cultures and others may feel it is inappropriate to discuss impending death with the patient, as they want to preserve hope.

- Buddhists may not want any drugs that cloud the mind near death. And some religions may teach that pain is part of God's plan, a test of faith or penance for past sins.

Food cravings are commonly experienced during pregnancy. The reasons for this appear to be at least partly hormonal, but there are cultural aspects involved, too. Women tend to crave foods that are available to them. In the Philippines, women often crave mango, while in North America, it is usually dairy.

Interestingly, many cancer sufferers describe cravings, too. My father-in-law had a burning desire for shrimp with seafood sauce weeks before he died. In our small town, there were not many seafood outlets. I went to the Chinese restaurant, got some fried shrimp, and made a sauce with ketchup and horseradish. This meal made him a very happy man.

Childbirth and death are by definition highly individual. However, along with personal belief, community has a powerful influence on the experience. As a physician or any caregiver, seeking out and understanding the rich backgrounds people carry will enhance the care we can give.

Obstetrical care and palliative care share a common thread for the practitioners. But what about society at large? Birth and death are the bookends of life. In every culture, in every country, we recognize and mark that with ritual.

CHAPTER 5

Rituals around
Birth and Death

No man is an island. No man stands alone.
—John Donne

Tokothanatology: There are many parallel rituals that deal with childbirth and terminal illness, rooted in history, religion, and society. Medicine itself has its ritualized patterns, especially in these two vital aspects of care. By examining some of the old and present-day customs and world rituals, we can see their importance in the study of tokothanatology.

THE BIRTH OF A CHILD CHANGES *EVERYTHING*—THE FAMILY structure, the hopes and fears and dreams of the parents and grandparents, the status of other children in the family, the mother's body, and even the father's body to a certain extent.

A death changes *everything*—the structure of the family, the hierarchy, the emotional connections, the financial state of a family, the sense of stability, the love given and received. All are disrupted.

We mark life events with rituals to give them form and structure and some guidelines to be followed. There are traditional ways to celebrate the birth of a child and help people deal with the death of a loved one. Knowing what is expected means the new family, or the bereaved family, doesn't have to make it up as they go along. Both family-centred maternity care and palliative care aim to be supportive of the customs that have meaning for people at these life-altering times. As caregivers, we need to be mindful of these customs and the fact that there are many personal variations in beliefs and practices.

Ritual involvement in childbearing begins well before pregnancy. For help with conception, ancient and modern fertility rites abound. Talismans such as the pre-Columbian sculptures I mentioned seeing in Elisabeth Bing's apartment are examples of the fertility symbols prominent in early art. Rituals and prayers were designed to help a woman get pregnant and to give birth to a healthy baby. Checking basal temperature or planning sex on certain days of a woman's cycle, although based on science, become rituals for many couples hoping for a child. Lynn Johnston has a cartoon in her first book, *David, We're Pregnant,*[53] which shows a couple talking. He says sadly, "This getting pregnant thing has taken all the sex out of intercourse."

The foods eaten before and during pregnancy can have symbolic aspects. In many early cultures, consumption of certain foods was encouraged to increase fertility and to ensure the healthy and safe delivery of a child. Throughout history, different cultures have held different beliefs about foods. For example, some promoted an animal-free diet so the child would not get the characteristics of a particular animal, while others suggested meat-rich diets so the baby would be strong.

Pregnant women are now advised to avoid alcohol, marijuana, and tobacco, based on good evidence, but restrictions such as these have some ritual aspects, too, since the mother is making personal sacrifices for the good of the unborn child. I did find a study done at the University of Helsinki, published in 2004, suggesting that

---

53   Lynn Johnston, David, *We're Pregnant! What's So Funny about Having a Baby?* (Stoney Creek: Potlatch Publications, 1975), 9.

mothers who eat chocolate during pregnancy have happier babies.[54] (I like that one.)

I saw many family members try to cajole a terminally ill loved one to eat, sure that eating would help them live longer or even recover. Refusing to eat can be seen as a symbol of giving up rather than a natural lack of interest in food in a weak, bedridden person. Sometimes, however, as a person nears the end of his life, preparing and offering their favourite comfort foods, overriding any previous dietary restrictions, can be a loving act.

For many years, women were not allowed to eat during labour because it was thought the food would go undigested, increasing the risk of vomiting. A review in the Cochrane Collaboration identified "no benefits or harms of restricting foods and fluids during labour in women at low risk of needing anaesthesia [...]. Thus, given these findings, women should be free to eat and drink in labour, or not, as they wish."[55] Still, many hospitals routinely send clear fluid trays to obstetrical units.

Fasting is a common practice among South Asians such as Hindu and Sikh people as they approach death. The fasting is thought to spiritually strengthen the person and bring good luck to the family.

From the beginning of time, babies were fed at their mother's breast or occasionally by a "wet nurse," a woman who was hired to breastfeed the child. Breastfeeding in the Western world declined significantly from the late 1800s to the 1960s. By the 1950s, breast-feeding was felt to be something practiced by the uneducated and those of lower classes. We gave babies sugar water as a first feeding to make sure there were no problems with swallowing, and bottle

54   K. Räikkönen, A. K. Pesonen, A. L. Jarvenpaa, and T. E. Strandberg, "Sweet Babies: Chocolate Consumption during Pregnancy and Infant Temperament at Six Months," *Early Human Development* 76, no. 2 (February 2004): 139–145, https://researchportal.helsinki.fi/ en/publications/sweet-babies-chocolate-consumption-during-pregnancy-and-infant-te.

55   M. Singata, J. Tranmer, and G. M. L. Gyte, "Eating and Drinking in Labour," Cochrane, August 22, 2013, https://www.cochrane.org/CD003930/PREG_eating -and-drinking-in-labour.

feeding was seen as scientific, modern, better. A lot of money and research has gone into producing formulas that mimic breast milk.

Breastfeeding is once again seen as the best option for many reasons. Immune antibodies pass through breast milk, protecting the baby. Breastfed babies tend to have better digestion and fewer infections. The cost savings, safety, and ready availability are all positive factors. Women who have breastfed have a lower incidence of breast cancer. We encourage suckling immediately after birth to help with the delivery of the placenta. These days, women who do not breastfeed can feel vilified.

Rituals abound around movement and exercise, as well. Pregnancy yoga helps to increase flexibility and relaxation and is often suggested to pregnant women in Western cultures. Yoga and meditation can also be helpful for the gravely ill person, easing discomfort and anxiety.

Belly dancing has been taught in the Middle East since ancient times, to show women how to move their bodies to help labour and is said to be a form of hypnosis for pain control. Self-hypnosis and creative imaging, or "going to your happy place," are helpful both in active labour and for dealing with unpleasant sensations in severe illness.

During labour, people do many things to symbolically ensure comfort and safety for the mother and baby. In places as far flung as Ireland, India, and Siberia, family members set animals free, loosen their hair, or unlock doors to symbolize the removal of any obstructions during birth.

Near the moment of death, some Hindus may prefer to lie on the floor in accordance with an ancient belief that a connection to the earth makes it easier for the soul to depart.

Ritual has a place in preparing a woman for delivery. One, called Blessingway, has been a part of a number of cultures, including the Navajo Nation people. This custom is designed to help a woman surrender to the mysteries of labour and birth and give them strength for the ordeal. Just before a woman goes into labour, a ceremony is done involving symbols such as eggs, beads, chocolate, and candles. Prayers such as this one are to be spoken:

Powers of the East, the Air, the deep breathing of labour and
the first breath of the new baby, join our circle.

Powers of the South, the Fire, light of life and intensity of labour, join our circle.

Powers of the West, the Water, water of life and the waters of the womb, join our circle.

Powers of the North, the Earth, the direction of the ancestors and
Grandmothers who watch over women during birth, join our circle.[56]

Many people find strength in religious protocols during child-birth. Observant Jewish husbands will recite psalms while their wives are in labour. I found many suggestions for prayers by pregnant or labouring women on a Christian website.[57] Here is just a small sampling of them:

"I ask for your Almighty hand to hold and keep us as we carry this precious gift."

"Merciful Father, thank you that every good and perfect gift comes from you.
May I feel peace and security in your arms as I give birth.
May your love fill my heart with joy. May your presence be my strength when I feel pain.
May your word give me peace throughout this process."

"God of All Comfort, remind me that this pain is temporary and is leading to great joy.
Keep my eyes fixed on you. Give me the strength I need to keep going. I can trust that
you will bring me safely through this experience, rejoicing in your great gift of a child."

(Although I have also personally heard, "Jesus Christ! Get this thing out of me!")

And from the website *The Muslim Obstetrician and Gynecologist*:

---

56   The original source of this prayer is unknown to me.

57   "Prayer for Pregnant Women," Living Prayers, accessed March 23, 2022, https://www.living-prayers.com.

For a birthing mother, the prayer remains an obligation until the baby's head is born. It is usually a quick push after that to pull out the rest of baby—shoulders and all—and the woman has entered into nifás (postnatal bleeding), meaning the prayer is no longer incumbent upon her.[58]

This website includes prayers for each stage of labour and afterward. Traditionally, a Muslim man would not be present at the birth of his child, usually a female-only activity. I did care for a number of couples in my community who wanted to be part of their new Canadian culture, while honouring their own teachings. Sometimes the husband would accompany his wife during labour and leave during the actual delivery. I remember one time a Muslim man stayed with his wife through a long labour, leaving only to pray. At the time of the actual birth of his child, he stayed in the room, holding his wife's hand but with his back turned.

A spiritual leader or family member may pray before a death in many traditions. The Muslim *Talqeen* ceremony helps a person to be spiritually ready for the journey into death. People present are encouraged to share in prayer, while the dying person makes an affirmation of his faith. The dying person should not be drawn into any worldly discussions, but if he discusses any worldly affair, then the *Talqeen* should be repeated.[59]

Prayers may be spontaneous and personal, but there are many suggested prayers to say at the time of death, such as this one:

"Eternal rest grant unto them, O Lord, and let perpetual light shine upon them. May their souls and the souls of all the faithful departed, through the mercy of God, rest in peace."[60]

58 Anse Tamara Gray, "Prayer and Labor and Delivery," *The Muslim Obstetrician & Gynecologist* (blog), May 19, 2013, https://www.muslimobgyn.com/prayer-and-labor-and-delivery/.

59 "The End of Life: Exploring Death in America: Readings," NPR, accessed April 20, 2022, https://legacy.npr.org/programs/death/readings/spiritual/muslim.html.

60 "Eternal Rest Prayer," The Catholic Company, accessed March 27, 2022, https://www.catholiccompany.com/eternal-rest-prayer/.

In the Catholic faith, last rites are final prayers and blessings that a person receives before they die, to give spiritual comfort and a renewed faith that they will walk with Christ and meet their maker. Usually last rites are given by a priest, but in dire circumstances, others may perform this duty.

A nondenominational prayer I remember finding very moving when I heard it goes like this:

> *Be free, be strong, be proud of who you have been,*
> *know that you will be mourned and missed, that no one can replace you,*
> *that you have loved and are beloved.*

> *Move beyond form, flowing like water, feeding on sunlight and moonlight,*
> *radiant as the stars in the night sky.*

> *Pass the gates, enter the dark without fear,*
> *returning to the womb of life to steep in the cauldron of rebirth.*

> *Rest, heal, grow young again.*

> *Be blessed.*[61]

Until recently, having a baby was a risky event. Many mothers died in childbirth, and death rates for children under one year of age were high. Many customs have evolved to increase the chances of a positive outcome. Amulets placed near the birthing bed containing prayers for a safe delivery are part of traditional Jewish practice. Japanese *omamori* are colourful brocaded silk charms that have been used for centuries to protect babies and mothers and to bring good luck. They are now often seen hanging on cell phones, on straps of baby carriages, and in cars. Red bracelets adorn babies born into Latin American families to ward off misfortune or *"mal de ojo"*—the

---

61   "10 Funeral Prayers and Blessings," *Funeral Guide* (blog), January 15, 2018, https://www.funeralguide.co.uk/blog/funeral-prayers.

evil eye. Red string bracelets or ties on a crib are popular in many cultures as symbols of protection. Red strings worn as a bracelet or around a person's waist are seen for dying people, as well.

Talismans also play a role after a death. It is common for a widow to wear an article of her late husband's clothing to keep something of him close. Many of my patients described keeping jewellery, a piece of art, or furniture that belonged to a family member for the same reason. A lock of a deceased person's hair kept in a piece of jewellery was a common memento during Victorian times. These keepsakes are symbols for those left behind, to help them go on with life while remembering the dead. And how many parents have kept a lock of their baby's first haircut as a memento of that sweet baby time?

The customs around dying for Indigenous people vary greatly. Many have Christian backgrounds; and many, when faced with terminal illness, will be comforted by some traditional practices, as well. Because the relationship to the land and nature is felt to be so important, dying close to home and their own community is preferred to hospital if at all possible. The importance of community and relationship in Indigenous communities flies against the rules that many hospitals impose. Hospitals may have restricted hours and allow just two visitors at a time. Often, though, medical needs can only be accommodated by admission to a hospital. Doug, as palliative care director in our hospital, would take on the role of traffic cop for his Indigenous patients, balancing the frequent visitors with the needs of other patients and with hospital policies.

Traditions around visiting the seriously ill are plentiful in most cultures, old and new. Buddhists feel it is vital to ensure a calm state of mind as a person is dying, so quiet visits and meditation are essential customs during that time. A Maori custom suggests that it is beneficial to visit a person before he dies, to establish a contact with their spirit which continues to exist after death. Having a spiritual leader, pastor, priest, or rabbi visit is important to many people.

Most hospitals have policies about visitors for a woman in labour, although some have eased the rules and leave it up to the mother herself. One of the arguments for a home birth is for the ability to have the people the woman wants in attendance, including her other children. A cautionary note here: whether at home or in a hospital, it is essential to have an adult present whose primary responsibility is the physical and emotional well-being of these children so the birthing woman is not distracted.

Many cultures encourage chanting or singing as part of the dying process. Offering a private area so this can be done without disturbing others can be a supportive gesture. There is a Buddhist practice of whispering one of the names of Buddha in a person's ear, or placing a piece of paper with the name in the dying person's mouth. It is tradition in Judaism that a dying person should not be left alone, so someone stays with her, reading psalms and saying prayers. And in some cultures and for some people, privacy in order to prepare for death is valued, so being aware and sensitive to this need can show respect to the person.

An experienced OB nurse can often tell what stage of labour a woman is in just by listening, even from outside of the labour room. The sounds of the breathing, the amount of chatting between contractions, the moaning or calling out, and the grunting sound of pushing can tell a great deal. (If the mother has an epidural, of course, this may not be the case.) However, there are external factors, as well. Some cultures expect the labouring mother to be quiet and stoical, while others expect a noisy affair of cries and grunting. I have heard some patients say they cry out even if they have an epidural so that the baby will be strong. Japanese women tend to labour in silence and give birth with very little pain medication, as the labour pains are said to help in the preparation for the challenge of parenting.

Before a baby is born, nesting is a ritual; many women feel a burst of energy and a desire to clean and organize the house in preparation for the baby's arrival. Another lovely custom involves designing a feng shui nursery, choosing the best placement for the crib and the most calming colours. Similarly, having personal items, photos, or music available in a palliative room can be a calming and supportive gesture.

"Lying-in" and "confinement" are two terms often used in relation to pregnancy. These terms describe the practice of keeping a woman out of society for a time before and after the birth of her child. There are many positive aspects to this practice: a time for a woman to rest and prepare before her baby is born, and later, a chance for her to get to know her newborn and to prepare for her new role as a mother, along with physical recovery and rest. The history of lying-in, however, comes from the idea that women were felt to be contaminated by pregnancy and birth, which was seen to be unclean and messy. In certain times, perhaps it also was used to avoid the obvious signs of sexual activity.

Different cultural groups have different customs suggesting how long this period of isolation should be and how it should look. The concept of a "fourth" trimester, the transition period after a baby is born, is often seen as a time of family-oriented isolation and nurturing.

After a person dies, some cultures advise a period of isolation for the bereaved, avoiding parties and social events, and a gradual re-entering into society.

Jarem Sawatsky wrote a book called *Dancing with Elephants*.[62] He suffers from Huntington's chorea, an invariably fatal neurological disease. The author had an unusual approach to revealing his fate. He and his wife decided to hold a big party and announce his diagnosis to their close friends and family. He decided that it was always better to celebrate than to mourn, always better to laugh than to cry.

Most people don't celebrate when they learn they have a terrible disease or that they are going to die. Generally, in the society I am part of, we keep this news quiet, suffering in silence, or at least within only our close circle. It is as if we are ashamed of the fact that we will die or suffer, and it's not OK to ask for help.

People do help and do step forward at times like this. Often, though, people shy away from the dying and their families and

---

62   Jarem Sawatsky, *Dancing with Elephants: Mindfulness Training for Those Living with Dementia, Chronic Illness or an Aging Brain* (United Kingdom: Red Canoe Press, 2017).

don't know what to say, so they don't say anything. There is a dis-comfort in confronting death, almost as if it is contagious, even when it's not. Having to face a dying person is an admission that we, too, will die.

I Don't Know What to Say, by Robert Buckman,[63] is a useful resource book with practical suggestions on how to talk to dying people and their loved ones.

There are rituals around announcing a pregnancy to the world. Whether to go public as soon as there is a possibility of a pregnancy or wait until the risk of miscarriage is lower is a decision each preg-nant woman and her partner must make. When to share the news may be based on family tradition. It may involve telling family at a special gathering or making sure family is informed before an an-nouncement goes out on social media. For some women, ordering ginger ale instead of a cocktail might be a way to tell her girlfriends she is expecting.

After the baby is born, people share the news with loved ones through phone calls, birth announcements in the newspaper, cute pictures in announcement cards, or now via social media. In my rural community, we sometimes see coloured balloons or handmade signs tied to the mailbox, announcing the birth of a baby boy or girl.

And we have many ways of announcing a death to the world. A newspaper obituary is the most common means of reporting, and traditionally, a family member will phone close friends and family after a death occurs. But more and more, funeral home websites and social media are used to convey the sad news and announce funeral arrangements.

There have been many superstitions around determining the sex of a baby before it is born. Many of these still exist today, if only for entertainment. "If the baby is lying high, it's a girl." "If the heartbeat is over 140, it's a boy." "If a gold ring is suspended on a string or the father's hair over the bump, and it moves in a circle, it's a girl. If it moves side to side, it's a boy."

---

63   Robert Buckman, *I Don't Know What to Say* (Toronto: Key Porter Books, 1988).

And then there was the Drano test. "If the mother's urine, mixed with liquid Drano, turns green, it's a boy. If brown, it's a girl."

That one almost had me. My patients began coming in with the results of their "Drano test" in the early 1990s. They claimed that they had done the test with their urine and that the baby was predicted to be whatever.

I decided to play a little game. Every time this information was shared with me, I would write it on their chart. And after the baby was born, we would see if it was right. Well, the first baby I delivered with the "result" on the chart was a girl. Bingo! Drano test agreed.

The second one, a girl. Yes! The Drano test had predicted a girl. And the third one was accurately predicted as male.

This continued for at least the next three or four deliveries. I thought to myself that maybe something crossed the placenta to the mother's urine that we didn't know about. Maybe there was something to the Drano test!

And then the next five deliveries disproved the theory; they were all wrong. But it gave me and my patients a good laugh.

Now, with the advent of our nearly universal access to ultrasound, predictions are most often accurate. And it seems more and more frequently, couples are choosing to learn in advance of delivery what to expect, so they can buy the right clothes, choose a name, or maybe begin to identify this little being as a real person. Gender-reveal parties are now common in many communities. The sex of the baby shown in the ultrasound is reported to the caregiver but not to the parents. The doctor or midwife is asked to reveal the baby's sex to a baker, so a cake interior can be baked pink or blue, or to a friend of the couple who will arrange coloured balloons, or even fireworks in the "appropriate" colour. I used to think that one of the things that helped a woman during labour was the anticipation of the reveal. Or maybe it was just my own anticipation of being able to declare, "*It's a boy!!!!*" My own little ritual.

At the time of death, a person's eyes are sometimes closed by an attendant or family member. The face may be covered with a sheet. Folklore tells of the need to cover the eyes so the soul is prevented from returning to the body. It is also felt to be a sign of respect for the body of the deceased. It marks the finality of death, making the person invisible. A friend described the moment her father died. "The doctor simply covered his head with the sheet and walked out. I wasn't ready to say goodbye. It was too soon, too sudden to acknowledge he was gone. For the doctor, it was as if my father wasn't important any longer."

Families may need some quiet time after their loved one dies, to sit with the body. Allowing this can be a kind and supportive gesture, whether before or after a professional has confirmed the death. Once the rituals begin—pronouncing death, documentation, making phone calls, etc.—it can be a very busy, disruptive time.

Last conversations with a dying loved one can form powerful memories. And a person's last words can take on meaning. Some "famous last words" have been immortalized.

Bob Marley said, "Money can't buy life."[64]

Sir Winston Churchill's last words were "I'm bored with it all."[65]

Goethe is said to have proclaimed: "More light!"[66]

According to Steve Jobs' sister Mona, the Apple founder's last words were "Oh wow. Oh wow. Oh wow."[67]

And my own Uncle Roy looked up, said, "Fuck it," pulled the covers over his head...and died.

As a parallel, I think of the importance we place on a baby's first smile, first words, and first steps.

---

64   Jane Lavender, "Bob Marley's Heartbreaking Final Words to His Son as He Lost His Battle against Cancer," *The Mirror*, May 21, 2020, https://www.mirror.co.uk/3am/celebrity-news/bob-marleys-heartbreaking-final-words-22051486.

65   Sarah Pruitt, "Famous Last Words: 9 Icons and Their Apparent Final Thoughts," *Biography*, last modified June 4, 2020, https://www.biography.com/news/famous-last-words.

66   George Henry Lewes, *The Story of Goethe's Life* (Boston: James R. Osgood and Company, 1873), 406.

67   Sam Jones, "Steve Jobs's Last Words: 'Oh Wow. Oh Wow. Oh Wow,'" *The Guardian*, October 31, 2011, https://www.theguardian.com/technology/2011/oct/31/steve-jobs-last-words.

Community customs such as giving gifts, having baby showers, and providing childcare for older children help after a baby's arrival. Rituals vary widely around when and how to visit. Some people delay taking the baby out, to avoid infection. For others, taking the baby to see relatives or friends is important early on. A coworker's visit to our office with her newborn on her way home from the hospital was a lovely gesture and one I remember fondly.

They say that "grief shared is grief diminished." After a death in a family, visiting and keeping in contact take on new meaning. Funerals, visitations, and sitting *shiva* are all customs aimed at providing community support to the bereaved. As with the gatherings around a birth, food and conversation are part of these rituals.

Rituals help new parents navigate the many changes in their daily lives once a baby arrives. They encourage support from family and friends and involve the community in celebrating the birth of a new member of society. Many of these rituals have a religious basis, blessing, protecting, and imparting certain characteristics to the child.

Christianity has its baptism and the naming of godparents for the child. Christenings are ceremonies of naming the child and introducing her to the church. In Judaism, it's the bris or ritual circumcision of boys, a covenant with God.

There are many fascinating ways that newborn children are greeted around the world. Muslim tradition has a ceremony in which the baby's head is shaved, to show the baby is a servant of Allah. The hair is weighed, and an equivalent weight in silver is donated to charity. A Muslim father whispers a prayer into a newborn's ear so the first word he hears is a prayer to Allah. Hindus may also shave the newborn baby's head to remove negativity from past lives, and some may pierce a baby's ears to ward off evil.

The practice in India, Egypt, many Asian cultures, and as part of an Islamic tradition is to place a bit of honey in a new baby's mouth, so the child will be sweet.

Many religions give guidelines on what is required after a death—specific prayers at certain times, when to see other people, what to do—giving structure to mourning. Having a very clear protocol means that no decisions have to be made during a difficult time. The idea that these same rituals have been practiced for generations gives a sense of community and purpose.

Jewish law requires that the person be buried as soon as possible after death, and psalms are read by the side of the body until burial, just as psalms are read during labour and at the bedside of the dying person. After the burial, the family stays at home for a week, sitting *shiva*. Friends and relatives visit the family home, sharing stories and prayers. Friends bring prepared food to the family for the week so they don't have to cook. Most communities have rituals that involve bringing meals to grieving families as well as to the family of a new baby.

There is a strong tradition of accompanying the dead. In Judaism, the body of the deceased is never left alone until burial. It is considered a *mitzvah*, or good deed, to make sure a person's remains are properly cared for after death. Having someone stay with the body until it is buried is common in many other cultures, as well. Filipino tradition says doing so guards the body so that the soul cannot return.

Pallbearers fulfill this same tradition of accompanying the dead. It is considered an honour to be asked to carry out this task. The ritual of naming godparents for a newborn child is a similar honour. By including people beyond the immediate family, we are saying we share our joys and sorrows with a wider community.

Traditions and rituals have been part of cultures at the time of death and afterward since the beginning of time. Archeologists have found human remains buried with obvious ceremony in every culture. Even Neanderthals seem to have had special ways of burying their dead.

Jewish and Muslim dead are buried as close to the earth as possible— Jews in a simple pine box, Muslims wrapped in a shroud and placed directly into the earth. Hindus cremate their dead, as they believe it's the quickest way to release the soul and help with reincarnation.

There are cultural differences in how a baby is carried. Holding the baby close to the body is soothing. Elaborate sarongs, wraps, and backboards allow the parent to have use of their hands or to allow access for breastfeeding. Baby carriages and strollers can be a sign of prestige or simply a vehicle for transporting the child along with the many items needed to take care of her while out and about—and maybe some groceries as well.

Graves can be identified in various ways. We see markers that range from a simple cross, a flat stone, or an engraved headstone with details about the person—the dates of his birth and death—to a large mausoleum signifying the social status of the person or their family. Some include benches to allow people to sit and visit their loved one's resting site. The cemeteries in New Orleans famously contain above ground vaults, as the water table is very high, and the land is prone to flooding.

New Orleans funeral processions to honour the deceased are a fascinating tradition. Jazz musicians accompany the hearse, often pulled by horses through the city, with mourners and many others following. The music starts in a somber way but changes during the parade to jubilant jazz so that "when the deceased is laid to rest—or they 'cut the body loose'—the mourners 'cut loose' as well."[68]

Funeral and burial or cremation rites vary, but all cultures mark the death of an individual in some way. It is customary in my community to have a visitation at a funeral home, where people come and give their condolences to the family and view the embalmed body in an open casket, along with mementos and pictures of the person's life. Charitable donations are customary. These are often designated by the family based on the illness the person died from or a cause dear to the deceased. It is popular for some people, particularly if they do not have religious affiliations, to forgo the funeral for a celebration of life, often at a later date. Friends and family share stories about the person and commemorate a life well lived. The Irish custom of a wake (traditionally with the body in the room), to drink to the soul of the departed, is still common in Newfoundland as well as the old country.

---

68   "The Jazz Funeral," NewOrleans.com, accessed March 27, 2022, https://www. neworleans.com/things-to-do/music/history-and-traditions/jazz-funeral/.

Contemporary ceremonies may follow religious models, but they often have a personal flavour. A niece said in her eulogy for her beloved uncle, "I am finally getting the last word, Uncle Chris!" For a woman who loved ice cream, loved ones set up a sundae station for the funeral lunch. A funeral for a young girl who drowned involved a little speech from each of her school classmates. For my mother, who loved music and loved to cook, we had a celebration of life with an open mic, so friends and family provided a concert along with tributes. We cooked and served all of her favourite recipes, from chopped liver to blondies. And after my father died, we spread both of our parents' ashes into the ocean and watched as the current swirled the two ash trails together. A lovely tribute to a marriage of seventy-two years.

I tried to attend the visitation or the funeral for my patients when I could. The family invariably expressed their thanks for the care I provided to their loved one. While attending these funerals was partly to support the family, I have to admit it was also partly to give me some closure and allow me to hear this praise. I often learned things about a person that I wished I had known during their lives.

For many of us, there is not much in the way of guidance on how to behave after the funeral, and people are left to figure it out on their own. As caregivers, we should be aware that grief work takes many forms and takes time. Coping through the use of tranquilizers or antidepressant medication simply delays feelings and is not often helpful. Many people express the fear that they are going crazy and are reassured when told this is not so; grief is a normal process.

New parents may also feel they are going crazy and need reassurance that they are normal. After a birth, the impact of this cute but oh-so-demanding human being and the feelings that go along with that can be overwhelming to the new parents. So are the physical demands, the sleepless nights, and the learning required to understand the language of the baby's cries.

Practices differ in different cultures and religions, but every group has guidelines for public mourning after a death; Latinos view crying as a sign of respect at funerals, while Tibetan Buddhists see it as a disruption. The practice of flying flags at half mast is a sign of mourning for public figures.

And many people have private rituals that help them through this time, from visiting places they associated with their loved ones to leaving a place at the dinner table. For me, taking over the task of filling the bird feeders in our yard was a ritualized way of dealing with the loss of my husband.

Gift-giving is common around a birth or death. For a new baby, it might be presents based on something the parents are passionate about, whether it's a baseball team, a feminist ideal, or Black Lives Matter. For the recently bereaved, it is more likely to be food, a planted tree, or a charitable donation in the person's memory. Baby books, which chronicle the child's "firsts" are ritual gifts, while guest books at visitations are common at funeral homes. And the ubiquitous Hallmark cards are used both to welcome babies and express sympathy.

Modern day Greeks put money into the crib of a newborn baby when they come to visit. This gesture is said to bring luck to the giver and ensure that the child will have a prosperous life. And Filipinos offer the baby money when the new family comes to visit, giving the homeowner good luck.

It is also customary to put money into a man's coffin during a visitation at a Greek funeral to help the widow financially, according to a friend of mine. She told me a story about a relative's funeral. My friend's son was a toddler at the time, and he reached in and grabbed some of the money before her husband could stop him. She was mortified! In Singapore, there is a custom of leaving bereavement money on a table in the funeral home to help pay the cost of the funeral—usually amounts that are odd numbers—as funerals are not auspicious events. The Irish custom of putting a penny in the coffin is to pay the way to the afterlife, as is the custom of placing coins on a deceased person's eyes or in the mouth.

In many cultures, there are standards about how long a person remains in mourning. These can vary from a few days to a whole year, although how long an individual actively grieves is a highly

personal thing. The behavior expected during the mourning period
can range from absolute rules to subtle guidelines, depending on
the cultural norms of the group. For some, dressing in black and
avoiding parties or gatherings are fundamental to their transition
time. For others, getting back to work and out with people may be
the way forward. It is important to reassure a person that everybody
grieves in their own way and their own time.

I have already mentioned that mothers often stay away from
society for a period of time after the birth of their child. There are
also many different customs about when to take the baby out into
the community, how the baby should be carried or wrapped, and
who will be involved in their care.

Birthdays are almost universally celebrated. A person's birthday
is his own, a reminder of his importance as an individual and his
progress through life. Birthdays, especially at cardinal years, mark
significant milestones worthy of celebration. Many people have
private rituals they carry out on significant dates after a loved one
dies—her birthday, an anniversary, Christmas, or the anniversary
of her death.

Many cultures have ways of remembering their dead, especially
on the anniversary of death. Catholics light candles in memory of
loved ones. Jews say the *kaddish* prayer and light a candle on the anniversary of a death. People may visit the gravesite and lay flowers
or objects significant to the loved one's life. Toys are often seen on
the graves of children who have died. Windchimes are a common
memento in cemeteries. We also see crosses near the side of the
road at sites of fatal accidents.

These tokens are ways of remembering and perhaps communicating with the deceased. My own mother explained why she preferred cremation for herself. She did not feel the need to have a
grave for us to visit. She talked to her parents and other loved ones
regularly. "I think of them with practical communication," she said.

Jizo statues representing "water children," or babies that were
not born, are seen throughout Japan. *Jizo* is the Shinto god who
protects children and the souls of children who died before their

parents. These statues look like children, often with red caps or baby bibs, as red is the colour of protection. There is an annual festival to acknowledge grief for these lost children, and parents often leave toys or snacks at the bases of these little statues. The grief associated with miscarriage, stillbirth, and abortion is not commonly acknowledged here in North America, but perhaps some kind of ritual could be adopted.

There are many other parallels in the customs we find at both ends of life. There is a lot of symbolism in colours. Black means mourning in much of the world. In much of Asia and in Indigenous Australia, white is the colour that signifies death; and in Egypt and Mexico, it is yellow. The almost ubiquitous pink for baby girls and blue for boys seems to be largely a marketing principle dating from the 1950s. Even that carries a lot of emotional undertone now, with considerations for gender equality and more acceptance of gender fluidity.

Water plays an important role at life's extremes. Spending part of labour in water has been shown to reduce stress and help ease the pain of contractions for the mother, and many birthing suites now include tubs. Bathing the baby soon after birth, along with providing a warm, quiet, dimly lit environment eases the transition from fetus to newborn, according to Dr. Frédérick Leboyer, author of *Birth Without Violence*.[69] He suggested we should view birth from the point of view of the child and make it a calm, welcoming experience. Teaching parents how to give the baby a bath in the early days is done to impart this parenting skill, but it's also a lovely ritual, allowing them to gently support and hold the baby, cupping his head and gently swishing warm water over him. Babies seem to relax and love this experience.

Infant baptism uses water to symbolically confer the beliefs of the parents onto the child in most Christian faiths. Sprinkling water on a newborn's head is a ritual way of inviting a child into the church family and is the first sacrament in the Catholic church, purifying the baby from original sin.

---

69   Dr. Frédérick Leboyer. *Birth without Violence* (New York: Healing Arts Press, 1974).

The act of bathing the dead has existed as a tradition from the days of ancient Egypt. Bathing and laying out a body after death can be a ritual way of showing affection for the person, caring for him as if he were a child again. Many religions see cleaning the body as a way of purifying the soul for the afterlife. In Hinduism, any river is considered holy. Some families will take their loved ones out of hospitals on their deathbeds to rest on the bank of a river, as it is believed that taking your final breath at the riverbank is the most beautiful way to die.

When my father was dying, he was admitted to the hospital for symptom control. When it became obvious that he was not going to be able to go back home, the staff moved two cots into the room so the family could stay with him comfortably. Many years ago, he had championed "rooming in," the practice of keeping the baby in the mother's room rather than in a nursery down the hall. Tokothanatology. Families should be allowed to be together at the bookends of life.

In our practices, doctors deal with the same problems multiple times, and every physician develops their own pattern. This amounts to a ritual: their own way of investigating, telling the person what is happening, what will happen, and what to do. We have patterns for taking a history, patterns of writing notes, and patterns of investigation. In obstetrical care, forms have become a fill-in-the-blank kind of ritual, so we remember to take and record the blood pressure, the weight, listen to the fetal heart, etc.

I learned by experience to book an extra long first prenatal visit, encouraging questions—there are no stupid questions—and encouraging a mother to bring her husband and children to visits if possible. Children at prenatal visits are wonderful. They are sponges for information, and they always want to help. I had many young children "help" measure mommy's tummy and listen to the baby's heartbeat. A toddler once picked up the doppler machine and, using it like a walkie-talkie, she spoke to "her baby" through the speaker. So cute. I would often tell other parents about that during a prenatal visit. I would talk to their children about what it would be like being a big brother or sister and how they would be able to help by bringing diapers, by singing to the baby when she cries, or by sharing nicely.

Later on, I learned that involving family members, especially children, in the lives of my palliative patients was equally rewarding. Children are often excluded from visiting very ill people. By allowing them to see their loved ones, they can have a more realistic idea of what is going on; this can help with their grief work later on. And they can bring happiness to the dying in so many ways.

With my palliative patients, I encouraged them to bring a friend or family member to office visits. This practice was a big help in getting all the details right and providing much needed support.

As physicians and other healthcare providers, we have many tools to help communicate the status of our patients. These have ritualistic aspects in that they provide a shortcut for sharing information and making critical decisions. The Apgar score, first developed by anaesthesiologist/obstetrician Dr. Virginia Apgar in 1952, is used regularly in assessing newborn babies at one minute and five minutes after birth. Up to two points are given for each of muscle tone, pulse, response to stimulation, colour, and respirations. This score helps in deciding what interventions, if any, may be needed for the baby.[70]

At the other end of the healthcare continuum, the PPS, or Palliative Performance Scale, is filling a similar role in communicating the status of a palliative patient. First developed by Anderson and Downing at the Victoria, BC, palliative care programme in 1996, it has become a standard assessment tool around the world.[71]

---

70   Leslie V. Simon, Muhammad F. Hashmi, and Bradley N. Bragg, "APGAR Score," *StatPearls* (January 2022), https://www.ncbi.nlm.nih.gov/books/NBK470569.

71   F. Anderson, G. M. Downing, J. Hill, L. Casorso, and N. Lerch, "Palliative Performance Scale (PPS): A New Tool," *Journal of Palliative Care* 12, no. 1 (Spring 1996): 5–11, https://pubmed.ncbi.nlm.nih.gov/8857241/.

The most recent version, PPSv2, was published in 2001.[72] This scale gives a percentage score for ambulation, activity level, evidence of disease, self-care, oral intake, and level of consciousness. The score is useful in quickly describing the person's current functional level, for workload management and for admission to hospice programmes. It has been shown to have prognostic value as well.[73]

How we navigate our interactions with patients, and the standards and best practices we carry out on a daily basis, form patterns of behavior that have ritual qualities. I believe that these rituals are an important aspect of medical care, giving continuity and some guidelines to follow. Understanding this idea gives some perspective on how we work and communicate. However, sometimes these medical rituals take on a life of their own and outlive the evidence of how to provide the best care. We should be vigilant and willing to change when new information becomes available.

The shaving of pubic hair at the onset of labour to reduce the risk of infection proved to actually increase infection rates.[74] The now standard caesarean section delivery of a fetus in breech position has meant that the skills needed to do a breech delivery in an emergency setting (or by choice) are almost completely lost. Routine electronic fetal monitoring was introduced to discover signs of fetal distress. Studies showed, though, that routine electronic fetal monitoring actually increases the incidence of unnecessary caesarean sections.[75] Even after being shown to

72   "Palliative Performance Scale (PPSv2) Version 2," *Victoria Hospice*, 2001, http://www. npcrc.org/files/news/palliative_performance_scale_PPSv2.pdf.

73   F. Anderson, G. M. Downing, J. Hill, L. Casorso, and N. Lerch, "Palliative Performance Scale (PPS): A New Tool," *Palliative Care* 12, no. 1 (Spring 1996): 5–11, https://pubmed.ncbi.nlm.nih.gov/8857241.

74   J. Tanner and K. Melen, "Does Hair Removal before Surgery Prevent Infections after Surgery?" Cochrane, August 26, 2021, https://www.cochrane.org/CD004122/WOUNDS_does-hair-removal-surgery-prevent-infections-after-surgery.

75   Ruth Martis, Ova Emilia, Detty S. Nurdiati, and Julie Brown, "Intermittent Auscultation (IA) of Fetal Heart Rate in Labour for Fetal Well-Being," *Cochrane Database of Systematic Reviews* 2, no. 2 (February 13, 2017): CD008680,https://www.cochranelibrary.com/cdsr/doi/10.1002/14651858.CD008680.pub2/abstract.

cause more harm than good, these practices have continued in many hospitals.

Life-threatening illness has also had its share of treatments which have taken on ritual status. Standard treatment plans can sometimes lag behind the most up-to-date evidence, something to watch for. CPR may be carried out as a final medical act. In fact, if there are no clear DNR or "do not resuscitate" orders in place, professionals are compelled to carry out a resuscitation even when it is felt to be fruitless. It is true that in the case of a sudden collapse, or at the immediate time the heart stops, CPR is a lifesaving procedure. But even in a palliative situation, some families or professionals may have a tendency to push for aggressive treatment, with the idea that "everything that could be done was done." This can bring comfort for those around the dying person and alleviate some guilt around the idea of giving up too easily. It is sometimes difficult for families and doctors to resist trying to resuscitate, even when the patient has said she doesn't want heroics. Discussions about advance directives and DNR orders can be an important practice so that interventions are appropriate and follow the wishes of the person herself. And just because there is a chemotherapy available for a particular cancer doesn't always mean it is the best option for that person.

In childbirth, Lamaze breathing and relaxation techniques taught in birthing classes have ritual aspects. Having a pattern to focus on gives the woman a guideline, something to follow without having to think it out. So do the birth plans childbirth advocates have encouraged. We put hats on newborns and bundle them in blankets to avoid heat loss, or we encourage skin-to-skin contact with the mother, to enhance bonding and also to avoid heat loss. Both have symbolic ritual characteristics and are favoured by different groups.

Assuming a healthy baby, we have routines for when to do an initial examination of the child and for who holds the baby first. Often, an excited, flustered father would have his camera or cell phone ready to take pictures of his newly born baby, only to forget when the time came. After the baby was safely handed over to the mother, I would ask if I could borrow the father's camera so I could snap some baby and family pictures. Those moments can't be repeated. I saw a few of the pictures; mostly I just knew the parents had them as family treasures.

Practices we take for granted in hospitals now may quite possibly be seen as quaint or unfounded in the future. Things that were once considered radical innovations have taken on ritual status. One father, when asked how the delivery of his baby had gone, answered, "Terrible! I didn't get to cut the cord." This step his fellow dads had talked about seemed so important, and he was disappointed he didn't get the chance to do it.

Illness and death don't follow a usual pattern the way child-birth does, so a simple checklist or form doesn't work as well as it does with childbirth. The techniques, the routines are much more individual, depending on the illness, the stage, and the patient's personality, age, or emotional state.

Nonetheless, doctors do have rituals to guide them in the care of the dying, whether they realize it or not. As much as each patient's illness and the care they require is unique, every doctor, nurse, or chaplain has a routine, a pattern they use over and over again. This routine makes a difficult job a bit easier to do. Sitting down, touching the person, and eye contact when discussing bad news are all little rituals we use every day.

I remember well the sinking feeling in my stomach each time I received a bad result and knew that I would have to share the news with my patient. I would take a breath, read it again. I would swear to myself, or sometimes out loud. And if so inclined, I'd say a brief prayer. And only then would I pick up the phone and ask my secretary to call the patient to make an urgent appointment. I tried very hard not to give bad news over the phone. Sometimes it was the only option, and I guess I had different routines for that.

I would tend to say the same things when I had the patient in my office. "I'm sure you are concerned that I called you in about this result..." I would go over the findings, explain what they meant, and discuss what the next steps were.

My ritual was to ask what questions the patient had, and I would repeat and repeat, because bad news doesn't sink in very easily.

I would write or print out something for the patient to take away with them and write myself a memo to remind me to follow up with a phone call or a visit within a day or so, saying to the patient, "I'm thinking about you. I have your back."

Many people say they would much rather die at home in familiar surroundings than in hospitals. In order for this to happen, there have to be people willing and able to do a lot of the care, with the support of professionals willing and able to visit as needed. Many palliative care teams have made remaining at home possible, with nurses and doctors available by phone and for home visits. For others, stand-alone hospice facilities are an alternative to hospital care when death at home is not a reasonable option. Some family doctors continue to do housecalls, especially for their very ill and dying patients, but many do not have the time or the inclination to provide this service. Where we see our patients has a lot to do with our own rituals. In the not so distant past, general practitioners saw their patients at home as often as they did in their offices or clinics, especially when they were very ill. With our heavy reliance on testing and technology, visiting at home is now less practical and less common.

I took on the care of a sixty-three-year-old woman who was dying of pancreatic cancer because her family doctor did not do housecalls, and she very much wanted to remain in her own home. Her husband and grown daughters were caring for her, with the help of home-care nurses. They lived on a farm, a distance from the main road and quite far from my house. I had a Red Hat luncheon event in a neighbouring town one day and spontaneously decided to drop in on her, as the side road that led to their farm was on my way home.

The Red Hat Society, in case you don't know, is an organization of older women who get together, not with goals of doing good or fundraising but simply to have some fun. We dress up and share a meal and some laughs. Good for my soul. So I called this family on my way home and asked if a visit would be possible, not thinking for a moment about my outlandish outfit—a large, floppy red hat decorated with a huge bow and purple netting, a purple dress with lots and lots of bling, red shoes, and purple stockings. I arrived at the door, said a brief hello to her husband, who just stood gaping at me, and walked into the living room where my patient's hospital bed was set up. I sat on the bed beside her and asked how she was feeling and what I could do for her. She laughed out loud and asked, "Did you dress up just for me?" and told me I had done her a world of good, showing up in my Red Hat outfit. It just made her day—and mine, too.

Having a baby at home also requires an appropriate environment and support people to make it safe and comfortable. Studies have shown that home deliveries for women with low-risk pregnancies have outcomes at least as good as, and in many cases better than, hospital births.[76],[77] The comfort of having family close by, having their own bed, and having less intervention is an appealing option for some women. Many midwives do home deliveries, with backup support in hospitals if necessary. Most doctors find more comfort in having all of the technologies and safety measures readily available. At present, more than 98 percent of babies in Canada are born in hospitals.[78] We have worked hard to make birthing rooms in hospitals more home-like, hiding clinical equipment and adding nice furnishings. This has become our "normal," part of our ritualized medical care model.

There is another ritual I would like to discuss: the tradition of telling your own story. New mothers want to tell the story of their labour, their delivery and their baby, and each new skill learned.

---

76   Gavin Young and Edmund Hey, "Choosing between Home and Hospital Delivery," *The British Medical Journal* 320, no. 7237 (March 18, 2000): 798, https://www.ncbi.nlm. nih.gov/pmc/articles/PMC1117782/.

77   Ole Olsen and Jette A. Clausen, "Planned Hospital Birth versus Planned Home Birth," Cochrane Library, September 12, 2012, https://www.cochranelibrary.com/ cdsr/doi/10.1002/14651858.CD000352.pub2/abstract.

78   Wendy Stuek, " Home Birth: A Labour of Love Few Canadian Parents Are Pursuing," *The Globe and Mail*, December 18, 2013, https://www.theglobeandmail.com/life/parenting/ home-birth-a-labour-of-love-few-canadian-parents-are-taking/article16050641/.

They say women forget the pain of labour once they have their baby in their arms. I'm sure the memories are blunted by this new focus, but many women find it affirming and healing to talk about their experiences in great detail. Their partners tell the stories, too, for that matter.

My mother used to tell about a time she heard a speaker at a conference describing birth as the "gentle opening of a flower, allowing the baby to emerge." My mother retorted, "It's more like shitting a pineapple!"

Suzanne Arms interviewed my father, then in his nineties, about his thoughts and his influence on the natural childbirth movement. As the only doctor in a small town, he delivered his own daughter. He said, "I guess I think of birth as what I had with Nomi. First of all, she was my daughter, and she slithered into my arms and it was so beautiful. Just nice! I enjoyed it and I think she enjoyed it. She cried, but I think she still enjoyed it...A beautiful experience, certainly it was to me and she says it was to her."[79]

Sharing the story about a loved one's death is the same kind of ritual. Telling it over and over is part of the way a person makes it real to themselves, to put some sense into it. Telling the story, any story of a dramatic life event, is a way of committing it to memory, deconstructing the event and the emotional burden. Stories about end-stage tragedies, end-of-life joys, miracles, epiphanies, and deathbed confessions are abundant in literature.

In real life, these stories are every bit as dramatic, sometimes in their mundaneness. Daddy told the story of our mother's death so many times I can repeat it by memory.

"I held her in my arms. I kissed her with each breath. And after there were no more breaths, I kissed her again." This story was also included in the obituary he wrote for her.

Caregivers also have to find ways of dealing with the powerful emotions that accompany childbirth and terminal illness.

---

79   Suzanne Arms and Murray Enkin, "Murray Enkin, MD," An Oral History of Wellness, uploaded July 21, 2020, YouTube video, 00:47:49, https://www.youtube.com/watch?v=5kNJxJe_LPc.

Storytelling is one of the tools that is especially useful. Going over "the case" with colleagues is a way of sorting out feelings. It can help us gain insight and learn other perspectives. We find ways of dealing with these life events, not able to change the outcome but able to have a positive influence on the journey.

Having some awareness of the rich social customs and rituals surrounding birth and death makes us more able to support the people we are charged to assist through these times. Some of what I would like to do with this book is to give readers some ritual, some format to help ease their own discomfort in caring for a dying patient—and, by extension, the family.

CHAPTER 6

Portrayals of Birth and Death

O, I am slain! If thou be merciful, Open the tomb, lay me with Juliet.
—William Shakespeare

*Life is always a rich and steady time when you are waiting for
something to happen or to hatch.*
—*Charlotte's Web* by E. B. White

Tokothanatology: Our many forms of storytelling often feature birth and death, so important to the human experience. What we learn from stories and how they influence our work and our perceptions is vital to the study of tokothanatology.

GEORGE AND HARRY WERE GREAT FRIENDS WHO PLAYED ON the same baseball team. One time, after a game, they were having a beer and got into a deep discussion. "Harry," said George, looking into his beer glass, "I wonder what heaven is like."

"I guess we'll know soon enough," said Harry. "Let's make a pact. Whoever gets to heaven first will find a way of telling the other!"

"Ha ha! It's a deal."

In the fullness of time, George died. Harry mourned for his friend and thought about him often. One day, George appeared before him.

"George, old friend! I've missed you! How is heaven?"

"Well, it's pretty wonderful. I have some good news and some bad news for you. The good news is there is baseball in heaven."

"That's great! And what's the bad news, George?"

"You're pitching on Tuesday."

A guy calls the hospital. He says, "You gotta help me! My wife's going into labour."

The nurse says, "Calm down. Is this her first child?"

He says, "No! This is her freaking husband!"

We share stories about the important things in life in many different forms. Jokes like these are a short-form way of imparting strong feelings. Literature, the arts, and other media impart knowledge and emotion and help us find meaning more effectively than textbooks or lectures ever could. Birth and death are big-ticket items, and the arts are rich with stories about both ends of life.

In this chapter, I will share some examples and encourage you to think about the impact they have on how we provide care. In my own experience, fiction in particular can show more of the complex feelings people experience during childbirth and death, and these stories have helped me understand my patients and even myself on a deeper level.

Depictions of both childbirth and dying date back to cave drawings and are seen in every culture, from ancient Chinese paintings to modern-day movies, television, and social media. They show just how significant the two ends of life are to our image of life itself.

Archaeologists suggest that pre-Columbian sculptures of pregnant women were fertility talismans. The Egyptian pyramids were tombs of Egyptian kings, everlasting monuments, their artwork a way of leading the soul to the next world.

Botticelli's *The Birth of Venus* is one of the most famous paintings of all time. Birth scenes are seen in many paintings, often shown with springtime backgrounds, symbolizing the start of life.

Artists in medieval times often used pregnant loved ones as models for their depictions of the Madonna. Women were encouraged to view beautiful things during their pregnancies, particularly pictures of a pregnant Madonna, in order to ensure a safe delivery and a healthy child. Many artifacts have been found with pictures of pregnant women and healthy children on them, given as gifts to young women for good outcomes in childbearing.

Deathbed scenes were often painted, sometimes with a fiddle-playing angel of death figure in the background. Memento mori, reminders to "remember you must die" were symbolized by skulls, hourglasses, guttering, or extinguished candles and faded flowers, and portrait painters often included them to remind viewers of the brevity and fragility of life.

Mexican artist Frida Kahlo's painting *Thinking About Death* is a self-portrait, with the wrinkles on her forehead depicting a skull and crossbones. In ancient Mexican culture, death also means re-birth and life. She painted herself against a background of green leaves, a symbol of life. In *My Birth*, *Henry Ford Hospital,* and many more paintings, Kahlo depicted birth, death, and miscarriage poignantly and graphically.

Turning to the written word, interestingly, birth stories are much less often depicted in literature than tales of death, but there are some memorable moments.

From Mary Costello's 2014 novel *Academy Street*:

The pain struck at dawn…In the hospital foyer her waters broke. She looked down at her drenched shoes and began to cry.

That evening when it was all over she thought she had scaled Everest, stood at its peak, exhilarated. The next morning the enormity of it all hit her. She had brought forth life, rendered human something from almost nothing, and this power, this ability to create, overwhelmed her…She was not in her right mind. Her body had been riven open, pum-melled, her innards displaced. A disgust at her physical self took hold, at the engorged breasts, the bleeding. I am a cow, she thought. But cows are good mothers. [80]

And from *A Tree Grows in Brooklyn* by Betty Smith (1943):

The baby was born. It was a girl and a very easy birth. The midwife down the block was called in. Everything went fine. Sissy was in labor only twenty-five minutes. It was a wonderful delivery. The only thing wrong with the whole business was that the baby was born dead. [81]

Margaret Atwood wrote *The Handmaid's Tale* in 1985, and it is now an award-winning TV series. Birth is depicted graphically in this dystopian story of women controlled by the state. In one birth, the woman is all alone, with no help; in another, the woman is forced to give birth publicly, in ritualized fashion.

In Ian McEwan's *Nutshell* (2016), the narrator is an unborn child who hears his mother's plan to murder her husband with her lover's help. He was distressed to realize they were talking about his father.

The narrator goes on to describe his birth in great detail:

So it continues, wave on wave, shouts and wails, and pleas for the agony to cease. Unmerciful progress, relentless ejection. The cord unreels behind me as I make my slow way forward. Forward and out. Pitiless forces of nature intend to flatten me...For a stretch, I'm deaf, blind and dumb, it hurts everywhere. But it pains my screaming mother more as she renders the sacrifice all mothers make for their big-headed, loud-mouthed infants.

---

80   Mary Costello, *Academy Street* (Edinburgh: Canongate Books,, 2014), 99.

81   Betty Smith, *A Tree Grows in Brooklyn* (New York: The Trumpet Club, with permission from Harper & Row, Publishers, 1989), 59.

A slithering moment of waxy, creaking emergence, and here I
am, set naked on the kingdom…I'm amazed…My faithful cord,
the lifeline…dies its allotted death. I'm breathing. Delicious. [82]

Literature is also rich with stories of death and dying.

Shakespeare's death scenes were memorable, in *Romeo and Juliet,
Hamlet, King Lear, Macbeth*, and so many others.

I remember being so moved by Beth's death in *Little Women,*
Louisa May Alcott's story of a family of girls. Beth contracts scarlet
fever while taking care of a neighbour's baby with the illness. She
becomes gravely ill but survives, only to die later of complications:

As Beth had hoped, the "tide went out easily;" and in the
dark hour before dawn, on the bosom where she had drawn
her first breath, she quietly drew her last, with no farewell
but one loving look, one little sigh. [83]

In Terry Pratchett's series *Discworld*, Death is a main character. In the fourth book of the series, *Mort* (1987), Mortimer is the
bumbling apprentice to the character Death. He learns that what
happens to a person when they die is exactly what they believe will
happen. So if you believe you will go to heaven, there you are. If
you believe you just disappear, you do. And if you believe (as one of
the *Discworld* communities believes) that you become a potato when
you die, you might turn into a french fry if you were naughty, or a
mashed potato, surrounded by butter and cream, if you were good.

A Funny Kind of Paradise, by Jo Owens (2021), is narrated by a woman
in a nursing home, immobile and unable to talk. Her last days are
beautifully described in the first person, along with comments by
her caregivers. "Death is like labour. It's hard work!"[84]

---

82   Ian McEwan, *Nutshell* (New York: Random House Large Print, 2016), 200–201.

83   Louisa M. Alcott, *Little Women* (Boston: Little, Brown, and Company, 1922), 339.

84   Jo Owens, *A Funny Kind of Paradise* (Toronto: Random House Canada, 2021), 229.

The Bible and other religious texts have many references to birth and death and stories surrounding them.

Genesis 35:16–19:

> [16]Then they moved on from Bethel. While they were still some distance from Ephrath, Rachel began to give birth and had great difficulty. [17]And as she was having great difficulty in childbirth, the midwife said to her, "Don't despair, for you have another son." [18]As she breathed her last—for she was dying—she named her son Ben-Oni. But his father named him Benjamin.

> [19]So Rachel died and was buried on the way to Ephrath (that is, Bethlehem). [85]

1 Kings 1:1–4:

> [1]When King David was very old, he could not keep warm even when they put covers over him. [2]So his attendants said to him, "Let us look for a young virgin to serve the king and take care of him. She can lie beside him so that our lord the king may keep warm."

> [3]Then they searched throughout Israel for a beautiful young woman and found Abishag, a Shunammite, and brought her to the king. [4]The woman was very beautiful; she took care of the king and waited on him, but the king had no sexual relations with her. [86]

And from the Talmud:

---

85   Gen. 35:16–19 (New International Version).

86   1 Kings 1:1–4 (New International Version).

Rava said to Rav Nachman: "Master, appear to me in a dream after your death." He appeared to him. Rava said to him: "Master, did you have pain in death?" Rav Nachman said to him: "Like the removal of a hair from milk." The dream continues with Rav Nachman saying even so, if offered the chance he would not come back and do it again, because the fear of death is so great.[87]

Television is an influential medium. Depictions of births on television often look like this: the woman, well groomed and with makeup intact, covered in many sheets all pure white and clean, screaming. The doctor, crouched at the end of the bed, and a bunch of other people all yelling *push, push,* then a baby's cry, and instantly, a clean, swaddled baby is in her arms, smiling lovingly at the beaming mother.

And the death scenes in movies and TV are so often like this: the man, with a fatal illness or wound, completely coherent and perfectly groomed, is about to disclose where the secret papers are hidden. Suddenly his eyes glaze over, his head drops to the side, and the information is lost forever as he takes his last breath.

Or this one: there are bullets flying everywhere. The hero ducks behind a car or a boulder, jumps up, shoots, and ducks back down, unscathed. The bad guys are hit. They scream and die dramatically and bloodily.

Not terribly realistic. But these portrayals have a great influence on how we perceive childbirth and death.

Things have changed over time. Pregnant actresses in the early days of television were photographed to hide the baby bump with different camera views or strategically placed furniture—and, in one well-known series, a large teddy bear. Lucille Ball made history, working her pregnancy into the story of her sitcom *I Love Lucy* in the 1950s. Demi Moore's nude and pregnant cover photo on *Vanity Fair* turned heads in August 1991.

---

87 Moed Katan 28a, (Babylonian Talmud); see *The William Davidson Talmud*, https://www. sefaria.org/Moed_Katan.28a.24?lang=bi

Deaths have been shown on any number of television programs, some shocking, some just sad. Dr. Mark Greene, one of the main characters on *ER*, died of a brain tumour, listening to "Over the Rainbow."[88] In an episode of *The Sopranos*, Tony Soprano smothers Christopher after he is seriously injured in a car accident. Christopher's eyes roll back then gloss over as his final scene comes to an end.[89]

There is a famous episode on *Sesame Street* after the actor who played Mr. Hooper, the grocer, died. The authors decided to write the death into the story, using it to show death in a way a child could relate to. Called "Farewell Mr. Hooper," the episode aired in 1983. Big Bird learns that Mr. Hooper is never coming back because he died. He is very sad. Forgetful Jones feels unhappy, but he doesn't remember why; Ernie performs in a feelings pageant representing love; and Bert loses his paperclip collection and feels angry and sad. To symbolize the circle of life, Big Bird meets a new baby on the block.[90]

Call the Midwife, the popular BBC series based on the memoir of a London midwife in the 1950s, has many fairly accurate depictions of births. Other popular fictional TV series, including *Star Trek*, *Friends*, *Sex and the City*, and *The Big Bang Theory* include pregnancies as part of their storylines.

Pregnancy and childbirth show up often on reality TV. *My Baby Is Having a Baby*, *I Didn't Know I Was Pregnant*, and *16 and Pregnant* were on the television schedule when I checked today. These programs and

---

88   *ER*, season 8, episode 21, "On the Beach," directed by John Wells, written by John Wells and Michael Crichton, featuring Anthony Edwards, Alex Kingston, and Hallee Hirsh, aired May 9, 2002, on NBC, https://www.amazon.com/ER-Season-8/dp/B0025WWVUI.

89   *The Sopranos*, season 6, episode 18, "Kennedy and Heidi," directed by Alan Taylor, written by David Chase and Matthew Weiner, featuring James Gandolfini, Michael Imperioli, and Lorraine Bracco, aired May 13, 2007, on HBO, https://www.hbo.com/the-sopranos.

90   *Sesame Street*, season 15, episode 4, "#1839: Farewell, Mr. Hooper," directed by Lisa Simon, written by Norman Stiles, Joseph A. Bailey, and Gary Belkin, featuring Northern Calloway, Emilio Delgado, and Loretta Long, aired November 24, 1983, on PBS.

others give us a picture of what the birth experience "really is," although what we see in real life shares little in common with them.

The events that are filmed, of course, are the "interesting" ones, the dramatic, action-packed, complicated births. No one would be interested in seeing tedious hours of contractions every five minutes, with dozing in between, the hour or so of pushing, hair damp and messy.

Deaths are likewise depicted in dramatic fashion rather than the frequent reality of hours or days of a comatose, frail person, turned every two hours, with family sitting vigil.

TV shows such as *This Is Us, The Good Place, The Walking Dead,* and *Six Feet Under* give the general public a perception of how death happens. Again, not terribly realistic in most circumstances.

In the movie *Meet Joe Black,* Anthony Hopkins portrays a man destined to die. He encounters Death (played by Brad Pitt) and bargains with him to buy some more time, before walking over the hill, while fireworks celebrating the man's birthday and a life well lived light up the sky in the background.

Whose Life Is It Anyway (1978) was a Broadway play, made into a movie starring Richard Dreyfus in 1981, about a sculptor who was paralyzed from the neck down in an accident. He pushed to be discharged from the hospital so he could stop the life-sustaining treatment he didn't want.

And there is a lovely movie about a girl who grows up in a funeral home (her father is a funeral director), *My Girl* (1991). She learns about death and dealing with grief along with friendship and love.

In the 1994 movie *Junior,* Arnold Schwarzenegger plays a pregnant man. *Twins* (1988) is another Arnold Schwarzenegger movie, also starring Danny Devito, which portrays two men as an unlikely set of twins conceived in an experimental pregnancy. And *Juno* (2007) is a story about a pregnant teenager and her relationship with the couple who will adopt her baby.

I know of two older movies that dealt with abortion issues: *A Summer Place* (1959) and *Dirty Dancing* (1987). I'm sure there are others. Stories of young love, especially in the days before effective birth control, made for compelling drama.

Social media has opened up a whole new format. Everybody has become an amateur movie director, and portraying everyday life is now commonplace on Facebook, YouTube, Twitter, and TikTok. Showing ultrasounds of babies, showing actual births, and tragically, showing some suicides on social media has become part of our social lexicon. There is a well-known phenomenon of teenagers reaching out over social media to share their grief after school shootings.

These real-life depictions of birth and death can be just as influential as the fictional accounts we considered earlier. Another way we communicate difficult emotions both in fiction and in real-life accounts is through humour, sometimes with a dark edge. There are millions of one-liners, jokes, and comic strips about being pregnant and about dying. It's not easy to talk about these subjects, so we laugh about them. Dark humour helps us cope with what frightens us the most, caregiver and patient alike.

"Why do they put nails in coffins?"

"To prevent the oncologist from giving that one last dose of chemotherapy."

"I'm twenty weeks pregnant. When will my baby move?"

"With any luck, right after he graduates from college."

"Do you know what the death rate around here is?"

"One per person."

"Due to the Coronavirus, there is a huge shortage of maternity ward staff. It's a midwife crisis."

Maria went to the doctor. She told her friend later that day that the doctor had given her some pills that would make her feel great and that she should take them for the rest of her life. Her friend said, "That sounds great! Why do you look so worried?"

Maria answered, "He only gave me four pills."

And then there is the story about Moishe. Moishe knew he was dying. He was very weak and spent most of his time in bed, sleeping or thinking or praying. People came to see him, but mostly he could hear the women working away in the kitchen. And the smells! He smelled delicious wafts of all of his favourite treats. Cookies, babka, apple strudel with cinnamon. He thought he would get up and get a taste of all of it, so he made his way to the kitchen, savouring the wonderful aromas as he went. Finally, he reached the countertop where all of these dishes were placed. As he reached out to grab a piece of strudel from a tray, his wife turned to him and hit his hand with her spoon. "Psha!" she exclaimed. "Leave it. That's for after the funeral!"

Lynn Johnston's popular comic strip *For Better or For Worse* started with a series of cartoons about pregnancy, birth, and parenting in the book *David, We're Pregnant!* (1973). When she was pregnant, Lynn was my father's patient and said to him, "You need some cartoons on the ceiling, for when your patients have to lie on the examining table waiting for you." He encouraged her to draw them, and the rest was, well, history.

In her comic strip, Lynn Johnston wrote about her mother's sense of humour in her dying days: "Here I am, preparing to meet my maker...and I'm worried I'll have nothing to wear."

It's not just whole stories, but also words that tell a lot about how we express attitudes about birth and death. We often use slang or euphemisms in discussing these and other sensitive topics.

In Victorian times, a pregnant woman was "in a delicate condition." When Lucille Ball wanted to use her real pregnancy as part of the story line of her sitcom, the producers forbade her from using the word "pregnant." Some common euphemisms to say a woman is pregnant are that she is with child, in the family way, eating for two, up the duff, preggers, expecting, expecting a visit from the stork, has a bun in the oven, or she's knocked up.

That last one is interesting but sinister. It refers to a female slave who became pregnant. "Knocked down by the auctioneer and knocked up by the purchaser."

We also convey our discomfort about death in the euphemisms we use. When a person has a terminal illness, we might say they are gravely ill or that they are in a bad way. We use genteel phrases such as *passed away* or *at rest,* and irreverent ones like that he cashed in his chips, he's pushing up daisies, she has expired, bit the dust, kicked the bucket, or is on the wrong side of the grass, six feet under, or gone to the farm.

True story, many years ago, my young nephews came to visit us at our farm near Kincardine. They got out of the car and started running around madly. After a bit, they came over to me and asked where he was. "Who?" I asked. They were looking for their dog, Bongo! Bongo had died not long before, and their parents had said that Bongo had "gone to the farm." It took a lot of talking and quite a few tears to explain that, no, Bongo wasn't here.

You may recognize this bit from the Monty Python Sketch:

> 'E's not pinin'! 'E's passed on! This parrot is no more! He
> has ceased to be! 'E's expired and gone to meet 'is maker!
> 'E's a stiff! Bereft of life, 'e rests in peace! If you hadn't
> nailed 'im to the perch 'e'd be pushing up the daisies! 'Is
> metabolic processes are now 'istory! 'E's off the twig! 'E's
> kicked the bucket, 'e's shuffled off 'is mortal coil, run down
> the curtain and joined the bleedin' choir invisible! THIS
> IS AN EX-PARROT![91]

As doctors, we model our level of comfort or discomfort for our patients. In discussions about sex, euphemisms are common. But we learn to use straightforward language when taking a sexual history, to improve communication and increase comfort with the topic. Once we learn to say the real words without shuddering—penis, vagina, erection—it becomes easier to discuss these things with patients. When it comes to death, the words don't come easily, either.

Think of the word *cancer*. Everything goes blank after you utter the c-word. People treat it like a swear word, like the f-word and the n-word, horrifying and taboo. Saying the words—the plain, real words—reduces stigma and helps us and our patients come to terms with the reality of impending death rather than pushing for

---

91　Monty Python Scripts, "Dead Parrot," Another Bleedin' Monty Python Website, accessed March 27, 2022, http://montypython.50webs.com/scripts/Series_1/53.htm.

unrealistic treatments or goals.

When my husband, Doug, died, I tried to simply say, "He's dead." But I recognized other people's discomfort when I said that, and I sometimes softened it to "he passed away," although it still grated.

Widow was a term I found difficult to use. My pen just wouldn't hit the right check box the first few times I had to fill out forms. Even when talking to other widows, I would say, "We are part of the same club."

While it was difficult to use the words, it seemed important to share the stories. There is an old saying: "Grief shared is grief diminished." I mentioned the ritual of storytelling in the last chapter. I want to reinforce the importance of telling "my own story." Telling one's story is a way to clarify thoughts, feelings, and memories. And listening to people's stories increases empathy and acts as a kind of witnessing.

Most women—and their partners, as well, when I think about it—want to tell the story about their own delivery to anyone who is willing to listen. Giving birth is one of the most life-changing events a person undergoes, and sharing the story feels good. Writing about their experiences in a blog or journal are other ways for new parents to share.

Do doctors listen to these stories? Of course we do, as part of taking a history and in getting to know and understand our patients. We could likely do better.

There are many written collections of birth stories, ranging from the dehumanizing, traumatic experiences of some women to the transformative, lovely births of others. As part of the advocacy movement for family-centred care and natural childbirth, these stories were ammunition for change and were made public for that reason.

Stories are a significant part of the grieving process, too, with survivors telling the story of a loved one's final journey. The need to tell it again and again is real, and it's a common phenomenon in the bereaved. Doug used to say that it helped to make the loss real to the person, and I found that to be true for me, as well.

These days, as more and more deaths take place in hospitals and ICUs, family members are not included in the care of the dying in the same way, so the ability to know and tell the story is often lost.

There is another kind of narrative related to dying: the many stories of "near-death experiences" told in literature and by individuals. We see eerily common traits in these descriptions, including a sense of peace, a light, a tunnel, and often seeing a beloved person who has died. People may describe a sense of leaving the body and watching from a distance, sometimes witnessing the efforts to resuscitate them. They may describe making a choice to go toward the light or to be pulled back to this realm with the pain and reality of the catastrophic event that put them there. Many people claim to have experienced this phenomenon, dating back as far as the Middle Ages.

Sherwin Nuland, in his book *How We Die: Reflections on Life's Final Chapter*,[92] has a scientific explanation for the sense of peace people describe when they have been in severe, life-threatening circumstances. He recounts the time Dr. Livingstone (of "Dr. Livingstone, I presume") was caught in the jaws of a huge lion and felt a "calm beyond measure, knowing he was going to die." Dr. Nuland explains that there was likely a surge of endorphins, which explains the near-death experience people describe.

I personally had a similar experience to the one Dr. Nuland wrote about. No lion, but a near-drowning, just a few years ago. Doug and I had gone for a drive with a friend in our side-by-side ATV to run our dog, Kitt. Doug missed the turn around our eight-foot-deep pond, and we rolled into the water. I was pinned under the vehicle.

I remember thinking, *Oh. I'm under water. Oh, I can't move this bar off my chest. Oh, I guess this is how I am going to die.* No panic, no fear, just a sense of peaceful inevitability. And no light. I survived, thanks to the quick, heroic actions of our friend, who rolled the ATV off me

92   Sherwin B. Nuland, *How We Die: Reflections on Life's Final Chapter* (New York: Vintage Books, 1995), 133–135.

and pulled me to shore, then ran all the way back to the road to get help. He also saved Doug and our dog.

Dr. Nuland's explanation resonated with me. That's exactly how I felt at the time: calm, peaceful, accepting. Perhaps the lack of panic is the reason I didn't thrash around and breathe in much water. Makes sense to me.

As caregivers, we have a need to tell our stories, too. There is an emotional toll in dealing with a difficult birth or a complex palliative care situation. Taking into account the necessity to maintain privacy, we debrief by telling our patients' stories to colleagues in a closed, safe environment, or to close friends or family without disclosing personal details. Doug and I both worked in these intense life-and-death situations on a regular basis. One of the things we would ask each other was, "Do you need to talk about today?"

The official story must be told, as well. Documentation is a legal obligation at both ends of life. We register every birth with the government. Death certificates include information about the cause of death, and there are specific guidelines on what is acceptable to write on them. There is actually a government office that reviews every death certificate signed in Ontario. If there are any irregularities, the forms are returned to the physician to be corrected. I learned the hard way that "old age" is not a legal cause of death. Nor is "cause of death: life." I know. I tried. They sent the forms back to me.

Our patients are influenced by the things they see, hear, and read about. All of this can have an impact on what they expect in their own lives. And because reality is often so different from these depictions, it is important to discuss their expectations regarding childbirth as well as care for a terminal illness. Teasing out some of these ideas and helping patients learn a more realistic viewpoint can be useful, dispelling misconceptions and fears. For instance, labour is a much more drawn out, tiring affair than we usually see on television, and most deaths are quiet and calm, not dramatic or painful. By looking at some of the popular media portrayals, we can gain insight into assumptions our patients may have, use them as a starting point for discussion, and attempt to correct any misconceptions.

As professionals, we are equally influenced by what we encounter in popular portrayals. We are members of the same society as our patients, and we watch, read, and listen to the same things. In many ways, our perceptions and assumptions about birth, death, and life were formed long before medical school. And we have our own life experiences, our own pregnancies, our own losses.

Even when we have real work experience, whether delivering babies or doing palliative care, how these events are depicted can still affect us. In my head, I carry the stories I have read along with the real births and deaths I attended and my own personal experiences. They melded into a complex narrative of joys, sadnesses, fears, and accomplishments, enriching the care I was able to provide to my patients.

I can remember watching episodes of the TV show *ER* and yelling at the screen about a caesarean section done in the emergency room. It was just so wrong. I am sure many of you have had similar experiences. While we can discount the distortion of facts as simple creative licence, it is worthwhile to realize that many people will see these depictions as accurate.

My sister-in-law Eva, a doula, discussed feeling frustrated about some of the births on TV. Clients get the impression that birth is scary and dangerous as well as action-packed, and they are not prepared for the length of time or the boredom. I think that's true of deathbed vigils, too.

Our comfort level in depicting childbirth and death has changed through the years. Reality is not always as simple as it appears in these depictions, but learning from these stories enhances our understanding of tokothanatology. In medical school, we learn about health, pregnancy, illness, and death for sure. But what we *know*, what we internalize, is based on the world around us. As caregivers, we have seen the real events, but we are influenced by media and the arts just as much as our patients are. Being aware of this allows us to use our knowledge more effectively.

CHAPTER 7

Pain and Other Symptoms or It Hurts!

It's not that I'm afraid to die. I just don't want to be there when it happens.
—Woody Allen

Suffering is only intolerable when nobody cares.
—Dame Cicely Saunders

> **Tokothanatology:** There are many symptom control measures and techniques we use for women in labour that we can utilize to improve comfort in palliative care.

THERE ARE PHYSICAL CHANGES THAT OCCUR IN THE BODY during and after a pregnancy as well as when a person is dying. Many of these changes are uncomfortable; some are dramatic. I will not go into the clinical details about pain and symptom management here; there are excellent resources for them elsewhere. In this chapter, I would like to discuss some ways we can help to ease the suffering caused by the complexity of unpleasant sensations at both ends of life.

The perception of pain is multifaceted. It is a combination of the physical, the emotional, and the spiritual, along with the memory of experiences and the meaning for the sufferer.

Education has been proven to reduce fear, increase understanding of the process of childbirth, and give pregnant parents tools for coping. Even changing the word from *pain* to *contraction* is useful. Learning empowers the woman. She knows what to expect and has some tools to manage the pains. Oops. The contractions.

Similarly, understanding about the disease and what is causing pain can be helpful to the palliative patient. Knowing what they are dealing with allows the person to accept certain sensations and fight against others.

When physical pain is controlled, a person can be more open to dealing with the spiritual and the emotional. It also allows a person to spend time with loved ones, to reminisce, or to make plans instead of concentrating on distressful symptoms. Rituals and religious customs around death and dying, as well as around birth, are healing and protective. Prayer itself can have a role in easing suffering. For many, religion plays a part in life-changing events, birth and dying, even when it is not prominent in their everyday lives.

There are numerous nonpharmaceutical ways of coping with the pain of childbirth. Imagery is one tool used to take the focus away from painful sensations. What this technique does is reframe the connotation from pain to intense effort. Thinking of a contraction as a wave on the ocean, rather than having the wave hit you and push you under the water where you struggle and gasp for breath, you can imagine surfing the crest of the wave. Labour contractions generally last about sixty seconds, so it can also help some women to imagine riding the minute hand around a clock. Or one can think of the birth process as a long hike through rolling hills, as a metaphor for labour.

Imagery can also be useful for the seriously ill person. For instance, invoking a picture of the chemotherapy fighting the cancer cells could offer a focus and meaning for what the patient is experiencing. Imagining the medication cushioning the nerve endings can enhance the relief a narcotic provides. "Going to my happy place" is a way of saying, "I'm pretending I am somewhere away from this negative feeling." For some, it can be soothing to imagine what heaven looks like. I have heard many descriptions of heaven from my dying patients, as they vividly and confidently described where they were going.

Focusing on one thing can block another sensation. Pain can be very intense, so to ease suffering, it's important to find tools for changing the sensation from bad to neutral. Concentrating on an object in the room is a well-known technique during labour. Some women will bring in a favourite picture or object to look at during contractions. Having a beloved piece of art or a family photo in the sickroom can have a similar effect for the dying person.

I am a proponent of meditation and mindfulness. The ability to live in the present moment, to put things in perspective and enjoy what is here and now, can help immensely. I know when Doug was ill, he talked about going into his Zen mode to ease his suffering, and meditation helped me through the dark times of his illness and after he died.

Hypnosis has been shown to be effective in easing the pain of labour. With training and practice ahead of time, a mother can go into a relaxed state of self-hypnosis and have a more positive and relaxed attitude toward the contractions. Hypnosis can be a powerful tool in reducing pain and decreasing stress in palliative care as well.

For some, making noise, from moaning to grunting, or chanting to outright screaming, can be a tool for dealing with painful sensations. These sounds are often involuntary and automatic but can be culturally determined. As I mentioned earlier, a Japanese woman will most likely concentrate in silence during labour. But an Italian mother may cry out loud with contractions, even when she has an epidural. Similarly, different people will have different ways of expressing and sometimes easing pain out loud when they are ill.

In prenatal classes, a woman learns different breathing techniques based on the intensity of the contraction. Helping a person breathe with Lamaze-style breathing through any episodic pain can help a great deal. I have used it myself, for severe menstrual cramps and at the dentist. We encourage palliative patients to breathe through uncomfortable procedures for the same reason.

For a woman who has not had prenatal training it is fairly easy to demonstrate a lot of this during labour. Touching a tight shoulder will help her relax. Having her look at your face and breathe with you can guide her to use these practices even if she has not attended classes. I breathed with my patients through countless contractions, as have millions of OB nurses, midwives, doulas, and husbands. And I have taught many dying patients and family members to concentrate on their breathing and use deep breathing or panting while waiting for a dose of opioid to kick in.

Severe pain can cause a person to hold their breath. This is a natural reaction to pain but has been shown to actually increase the unpleasant sensation. So teaching slow, steady breathing for early contractions and panting for the intense, later contractions can effectively reduce the pain. And encouraging palliative patients to breathe rather than holding their breath gives them something to concentrate on.

Similarly, stress-related hyperventilation causes unpleasant sensations. The simple cure is rebreathing—having the person breathe into a paper bag or cupped hands. Doing this allows their carbon dioxide levels to return to normal and alleviates the symptoms. Counting breaths is another tool that can reduce anxiety. It can help a woman through a contraction or help reduce unpleasant symptoms in the palliative patient.

The technique of consciously relaxing the rest of the body as soon as a contraction starts is a useful one. I would explain to my patient that the uterus needs to work hard, and tensing up other muscles takes needed energy away. I would often see a woman with her shoulders up near her ears, her face tight during a contraction as a reaction to the pain. If her body is tense, pain is increased. So specific instructions to relax the shoulders, relax the face, or to smile can all help reduce the pain perception. Teaching her to do this in prenatal classes gives her and her partner another tool to use and provides a sense of control. Learning yoga before the birth also helps the relaxation and sense of control during labour. We can see how the same techniques might ease some of the discomforts of illness.

Fear of the pain of labour can increase negative sensation. Fear can make the woman resist the contraction rather than flowing with it, physically tightening her body and mentally anticipating the next contraction with dread. According to the principles Dr. Dick-Read explained, when the labouring woman understands that the reason for the contractions is to push the baby down the birth canal and out, it gives purpose to the pain rather than "What the hell was that, and will it ever end?"

Similarly, in cancer and other diseases, knowledge about what is going on can reduce some of the fear of the unknown and lessen angst.

How we perceive pain is a matter of much research and speculation. The Gate Theory is one medical model that can help define what happens.[93] It explains that pain and other sensations follow common neural pathways in the spinal column, so the perception of light touch or pressure can override a painful sensation, blocking the pain message to the brain. Techniques such as effleurage (a circular stroking movement on the belly with the palm of the hand) or massage are often taught in prenatal classes and make use of this phenomenon. Acupuncture works in much the same way. Endorphins are hormones that cause a pleasant sensation, partly by blocking pain receptors. They are released in response to exercise, laughter, and other activities and are natural pain reducers. It is easy to see that these techniques could be applied to gravely ill people in pain.

For a woman in labour, the caregiver's attitude as well as that of her support people is reflected in the woman's perception. A calm midwife will help the woman see her situation as progressing normally, while a look of panic in the eyes of the caregiver will be noticed and internalized. For the terminally ill person, the frame of mind of the caregivers and loved ones can have a powerful effect on the suffering patient. People are not easily deceived. Honestly sharing concerns, in a gentle way, can be much more comforting than false reassurances.

93   R. Melzack and P. D. Wall, "Pain Mechanisms: A New Theory," *Science* 150, no. 3699 (November 19, 1965): 971–979, https://pubmed.ncbi.nlm.nih.gov/5320816. See also Lorne M. Mendell, "Constructing and Deconstructing the Gate Theory of Pain," *Pain* 155, no. 2 (February 2014): 210–216, https://www.ncbi.nlm.nih.gov/pmc/articles/PMC4009371/.

Nonpharmaceutical pain control measures such as hypnosis, acupuncture, and meditation all have a place in the birthing room as well as the sickroom. Ice or heat. Change in position. Distraction. They work. They can lessen the sensation of pain or make it disappear. Music has an especially soothing effect, both in labour and for the dying. There is good evidence this is true.[94] Of course, people's choice in music varies. I remember one woman who chose heavy metal as her playlist—it did help her to relax, and fortunately, she was the only labouring woman in the department at the time. For many of my patients in palliative care, gospel music was soothing; for others, opera or country was the music of choice. When asked what a nice donation to his palliative care department might be, Doug would request CD players, or later, iPods with playlists.

As medical people, we sometimes find it difficult to support alternative ways of treating our patients. We should be mindful of different ideas or rituals during childbirth as much as possible. Medicine does not have all the answers in treating serious disease, either. There is science behind a lot of alternative therapies, and even where there isn't, if they help, then good! The placebo effect comes into play here as well. So when a patient tells you that an unusual diet or Reiki or coffee enemas are working for them, it is helpful to be supportive and try to keep an open mind. Potential adverse effects should be part of the discussion, but if you show some interest, people will be more willing to share the information with you.

I am cautious, though, about charlatans who are willing to take money for false claims and false hope. These people prey on the vulnerable. We need to think of family as part of the "patient." Bankrupting the family by misleading them—getting them to agree to expensive, untested treatments—and taking advantage of the belief that they must do everything possible to find a cure is un-ethical and damaging. I can remember a patient whose family took

94   David H. Bradshaw, Gary W. Donaldson, Robert C. Jacobson, Yoshio Nakamura, and C. Richard Chapman, "Individual Differences in the Effects of Music Engagement on Responses to Painful Stimulation," *The Journal of Pain* 12, no. 12 (December 2011): 1262–1273, DOI: 10.1016/j.jpain.2011.08.010.

her to another country to have what they called "magic surgery." The "surgeon" used no anaesthetic, no knife. He had the woman lie down on a table, reached down, said some incantations, and reached "into her" and brought up a bloody mass of tissue and declared her cured of her cancer.

My guess is that he had a goat liver or something like that in his hand. They returned to Canada, where she died from metastatic cancer. To pay for the "magic surgery," the family sold their home, their truck, and heaven knows what else. Even without the money issue, false expectations can be harmful.

I do realize my bias here. If someone wants to use a cultural healing practice, or a religious ritual, or any nonmedical way of treating the disease or the symptoms, who am I to say only my way is right?

Deciding what to treat and what not to is part of the decision-making in the concept of palliative care. So, for instance, if a person has pneumonia, is coughing terribly, and has shakes and fevers, it might be quite reasonable to treat with antibiotics in order to relieve the discomfort. But if she is just quietly taking shallow breaths and is not in distress, and has a terminal condition, the better choice may be to withhold antibiotics and "let nature take its course." The old saying was that "pneumonia is the old man's friend."

When a person has a terminal illness, we should avoid testing just to see what is going on. The routine blood work we order automatically—the ritual, if you think about it—can cause a significant amount of pain and distress. Having to move to get an X-ray can take a great deal of effort. So think. Before you order a test, think about how knowing the answer would change your behavior. If it won't, don't do the test.

One of the things bedridden people really dislike if they are in pain and immobilized is to be turned. It's uncomfortable and takes a great deal of effort for the staff as well as the patient. But not turning them leads to pressure sores, skin breakdown, and pain.

I have very few regrets when it comes to how I cared for Doug in his final months, but that is one. He hated being turned, and it was very hard to do. So I gave in and didn't insist. I was alone with him for twelve hours most days, occasionally twenty-four hours, and I had recently had back surgery. I guess that was a good excuse, along with the reluctance on Doug's part. But he did develop painful bedsores that increased his discomfort at the end of his life. I'm sorry, Doug. I should have pushed you to allow the turns and gotten some help to do it. So, following the principle of doing things only if they contribute to comfort, turning is a good one to do. But give pain medication before, not after, and explain.

Safety and risk are different in the two kinds of care we are discussing here, of course. In pregnancy and delivery, therapeutic choices must keep the safety of the baby as well as the mother first and foremost.

When dealing with a terminal illness, this is less of a concern. Worrying about addiction to medication is counterproductive. But one must consider side effects of overdose or consequences of surgery and chemotherapy in any decision regarding treatment options.

Treating any pain is possible, but it might be at the cost of drowsiness or even unconsciousness. In maternity care, twilight sleep, popular in the first half of the last century, was a combination of drugs which induced pain relief and removed the memory of the pain of birth. Unfortunately, it caused a lack of awareness and control for the mother, just like heavy doses of narcotics can at the end of life. The element of choice is important. A cancer patient may decide to hold off on his pain medication in order to have a clear conversation with a visitor, for instance. Or they may wish to receive enough medication to have complete pain relief and just sleep the time away.

The contractions of labour tend to come at regular intervals, so timing is built into the process. Projecting to the end of each contraction is a coping mechanism in itself. Each contraction is one step closer to the mother having her baby in her arms.

Timing plays a different role in the terminally ill patient who has pain. If we order medication "as needed," the person must decide when to ask for a pill and then wait for the nurse to bring it to her; by the time it takes effect, her pain may be much worse. Doug always talked about the analogy of a kitchen fire in treating chronic pain. If you have a small fire on the stove, a lid over the pot or a small glass of water can put it out. But if you wait, you need the whole fire department to extinguish the flames. Medication for persistent pain should be given at regular intervals, or "by the clock." This way, we can decrease the anxiety caused by anticipating an increase in the pain, a powerful fear.

Pain has different meanings in different contexts. We all react to pain based on this underlying meaning. Aching legs while running a marathon tells a person they are using their muscles to capacity. In childbirth, the contractions, while painful, carry the meaning that this is the work needed to bring the baby. When a mother understands the process of what her body needs to do, she is more able to bear the discomfort and use techniques to help. But the pain of labour can also trigger memories of sexual trauma or events from previous deliveries. Pain can be associated with fears such as uncertainty about her ability to parent well, and fear can increase pain, leading to the buildup of a negative loop.

In terminal illness, a similar circle of emotions has the potential to increase suffering. Pain can mean "I'm dying," which evokes a feeling of "I'm afraid," which causes an increase in the pain. Past experiences or stories of how others suffered in illness can influence the suffering a person experiences. Or even, as I discussed in the last chapter, what they have witnessed through media, literature, or art.

Being aware of this and spending some time discussing it, teasing out these feelings, can help caregivers understand their patients' suffering and so help ease the pain.

Eric Cassell discusses the idea of existential suffering in *The Nature of Suffering*[95] as distinct from the physical sensation of pain. When physical pain is controlled, a person can focus on important

---

95   Eric J. Cassell, *The Nature of Suffering and the Goals of Medicine* (Oxford: Oxford University Press, 1991).

things such as connecting with family, a life review, and enjoying the moment. At the same time, dealing with spiritual pain can bring relief to physical discomfort.

Having a meaningful talk with a chaplain or spiritual care practitioner, or really with anyone who is willing to take the time, can help a person find their peace. I have seen, over and over, how relieving the angst and minimizing the fear helps the physical suffering of a dying person.

It may seem that this is outside the scope of the family doctor. However, the doctor is often a trusted person, one with whom the patient wishes to share his deepest feelings. So when I go into a patient's room to do a quick check-in and they say to me, "Doc, I haven't seen my son in three years, and I'm frightened I won't see him before I die," the right thing to do is to sit down, look him in the eye, and say, "Tell me what's going on." If I brush it off, or ignore it, or say I'll be back later, the moment may be gone forever.

Human to human connection does not look at rank or role. I know for a fact sometimes it's a member of the cleaning staff who listens and offers support.

It is so important to let the patient set the agenda. It rarely goes well when the professional opens a discussion with "Today we are going to talk about your death, your anger, the meaning of life, whatever." You could be met with "Doc, I'm constipated. Can I have a laxative?" or "Get the fuck out of my room!"

Pain isn't just about the physical feelings a person is experiencing. When facing death, questions about an afterlife and wondering what will happen are very real. Unfinished business, family disappointment, and unresolved arguments all take on an importance, an urgency that may not have existed before.

We may also worry about loved ones who will be left behind, a grief for things left unfinished. We might encounter the emotional challenges of feeling useless, of being a burden, of the anger, depression, and other feelings that accompany dying.

Emotions have a huge impact on expectant parents, as well. Wondering how they will manage the job of raising a child, along with thoughts about family expectations or money, can shape how a woman copes with the discomforts of pregnancy and the intensity of labour and delivery. Worries about the health of the child or fear for the mother's safety during childbirth can create a different perception of the experience.

Other distressing physical symptoms can have a huge effect on a person's sense of well-being, whether for a woman during her pregnancy, labour, and delivery or for a dying patient. Simple remedies can really make a difference in easing suffering. We tend to dwell on pain, especially with cancer, but many other causes of suffering are very real.

Nausea, to many, is worse than pain in its ability to distract the mind. There are medications as well as herbal treatments that do help. Hypnosis is extremely useful in controlling nausea and vomiting. Research shows evidence that cannabis helps control the nausea that accompanies chemotherapy.[96] And while the evidence is not yet clear, many people are using cannabis for pain control, with good results.[97]

"Nothing matters but the bowels" is a rallying cry in palliative care circles. If the bowels are not working normally, suffering can be severe. Narcotics, often essential for pain control in severe illness, always cause constipation and so should always be accompanied by a laxative. Constipation is also very common in late pregnancy, with the baby's head pressing down and taking up all the room. So in pregnancy, too, nothing matters but the bowels. It goes without saying that for the pregnant mom, diets should be high in fibre.

---

96   Linda A. Parker, Erin M. Rock, and Cheryl L. Limebeer, "Regulation of Nausea and Vomiting by Cannabinoids," *British Journal of Pharmacology* 163, no. 7 (August 2011): 1411–1422, https://www.ncbi.nlm.nih.gov/pmc/articles/PMC3165951/.

97   Martin Mücke,Tudor Phillips, Lukas Radbruch, Frank Petzke, and Winfried Häuser, "Cannabis-Based Medicines for Chronic Neuropathic Pain in Adults," Cochrane Library, March 7, 2018, https://www.cochranelibrary.com/cdsr/doi/10.1002/14651858. CD012182.pub2/full; Sonja Vučković, Dragana Srebro, Katarina Savić Vujović, Čedomir Vučetić, and Milica Prostran, "Cannabinoids and Pain: New Insights from Old Molecules," *Frontiers in Pharmacology* 9, article 1259 (November 2018), https://www.ncbi. nlm.nih.gov/pmc/articles/PMC6277878/.

And diarrhea as a side effect of chemotherapy can be debilitating, so medication and dietary adjustments are helpful.

Shortness of breath is a distressing symptom. Simple things such as a fan in the room, along with medical treatment, can ease this dramatically.

Simple remedies can often ease skin changes, appetite loss, and fatigue. Rashes and uncomfortable skin conditions are common both in pregnancy and in late-stage illness, for various reasons. Pruritus of pregnancy (which can be caused by an accumulation of liver enzymes in the skin), along with other causes of itchy skin during pregnancy, are temporary but distressing. In cancer patients, radiation burns and skin breakdown due to tumour growth or malnutrition are common skin issues. Stretching of skin due to a growing fetus—or swelling due to fluid buildup, seen in many illnesses—can cause a feeling of tightness and itching. While it is important to treat the underlying causes, symptomatic remedies such as cool compresses, soothing lotions, oatmeal baths, and antihistamines often help.

Sometimes, bad odours occur with infections or when cancers break down tissue. They can be very difficult to cope with, for the patient and for the people around him. It is demoralizing when people avoid visiting because they find the odour disturbing, and for the patient, there is no getting away from the smell. Simple remedies are often very effective. Lemon-scented sprays, or even cut lemons in a bowl, freshly ground coffee, charcoal briquettes, or baking soda are natural substances which neutralize or absorb odours and are readily available. Charcoal dressings and other odour-absorbing treatments are useful in a palliative care setting.

In both the patient and the professional, there is a tendency to attribute all symptoms to the pregnancy or to the terminal illness. It is valuable to remember that other discomforts or diseases can still be at play.

My mother had breast cancer years ago. And don't forget, my father was a doctor. My dad called me a few weeks after her surgery, saying they were sure the cancer had spread. She had a burning pain down one leg, and now she had spots on her leg. "Daddy, she has shingles!" I proclaimed over the phone from 200 km away. And I was right. She survived that cancer and lived another thirty-some years.

I remember a pregnant patient we thought was going into premature labour, until we realized she had acute appendicitis. And the patient with bowel cancer who developed a painful lump on his leg. It wasn't a metastatic deposit. It was a thorn embedded under his skin from a walk in the woods a few weeks before.

Once a person has had a cancer diagnosis, whether life-threatening or not, the assumption is that any symptom from that point on is related to the cancer. It is worth remembering that other illnesses and events still can and do happen. I do want to point out that pain is not synonymous with dying. And not all terminal illness is painful. Discomfort due to many causes can and must be addressed. I have noticed that many people have the idea that once morphine is prescribed, death is imminent. Not true! Narcotic medications such as morphine are highly effective analgesics that are useful in many reversible circumstances.

We have seen that methods of coping with pain and symptoms of pregnancy and birth are in many ways applicable to the dying person. The pain control techniques of prepared childbirth education can be taught and used to help ease the pain of cancer and other illnesses. The emotional and spiritual discomfort of both are equally troubling. And taking the time to listen, to support, has a huge and lasting impact on the well-being of our patients and their loved ones.

CHAPTER 8

Ethical and Legal Issues around Birth and Death

Technology has removed the mystery of death and life.
It has created the illusion that death is optional.
—Cynda Rushton, professor of clinical ethics
at Johns Hopkins University

It's simple. Just do the right thing.
—says pretty well everybody

> **Tokothanatology**: Life and death questions are inherent at both ends of life, and the decisions made are often controversial. Ethical and legal factors affecting care around reproduction, pregnancy, and childbirth, and in the care of the dying, have many parallels, such as the rights of individuals and the need to deal with differences in opinion in constructive and fair ways.

A SIXTEEN-YEAR-OLD PATIENT IS IN MY OFFICE. HAPPILY pregnant. She is not sure who the father is. She sees her pregnancy as a means of getting away from her toxic parents and of having "someone to love her." And how does this scenario change if I suspect she is using cocaine?

A man in his eighties asks me to help him commit suicide. He has terrible pain from his arthritis, and he is lonely. He has had enough of this damned life.

A mother calls to say she will sue me if I give the pill to her daughter. The thirteen-year-old girl comes to my office later the same day, saying she is sexually active and wants birth control. What are my options when I sit down with the daughter? What are my legal obligations? My moral ones?

A family meeting reveals that my sixty-two-year-old patient with bowel cancer is refusing surgery. His son wants me to declare him incompetent so he can be forced to have the likely lifesaving operation.

A pregnant woman at just over forty weeks gestation has been in labour for eighteen hours and is not progressing as I would like. She is exhausted. The fetal heart rate is not showing any signs of distress. I suspect the position of the fetus is posterior and the baby's head is still very high. The nurses feel it is time to do a caesarean section. The patient refuses. It's up to me to make the final decision and deal with the consequences.

A woman with end-stage lung cancer tells me about a long-standing (and secret, she hopes) affair with a man—her husband's best friend. She thinks her daughter may be this man's child, but she isn't sure. She asks for my guidance as she lies there on her deathbed. Should she tell? And what if the daughter has a crush on the lover's son?

These are all true stories, all from my own experience. Doctors and other healthcare providers who care for patients at both ends of life face ethical dilemmas such as these on a regular basis. Everybody has strong opinions about what is right, and often in situations such as the ones I have described, the opinions can be very different.

The traditional principles of medical decision-making are:

- beneficence, or doing good

- nonmaleficence, meaning "do no harm"

- autonomy, or control by the individual

- justice, or fairness.[98]

We make medical decisions based on these ethical principles every day. Keeping these four basic tenets in mind when faced with a dilemma can often make the decision clearer and help the involved parties understand opposing points of view. Things are not always as straightforward as they may seem at first glance. In the practice of tokothanatology—i.e., caring for people who are giving birth, those facing terminal illness, and all of the people involved in their lives—conflicts are very real. Particularly at the extremes of life, moral, religious, legal, social, personal, and even financial factors intertwine to make the "right thing" a complex matter.

So take a breath before tackling this chapter. I will be looking at big questions about reproductive health and care of the terminally ill. This may open up some deeply held beliefs and some strong emotional responses. Worth reading, but please take your time with it, and keep an open mind.

Family-centred maternity care is based on these four ethical principles: give the best-possible, safest care to mother and baby (beneficence); avoid harmful practices (nonmaleficence); allow for choice in all aspects of pregnancy and delivery (autonomy); and assure these are available to all (justice).

At the end of life, the same basic principles apply. Provide the best and safest care available. Avoid treatments that will cause more harm than good. Have discussions about choices in treatment and the option of declining it, while still offering support. And ensure the best treatments and excellent palliative care are available to all.

Supporting a patient's decision to go ahead with treatment or decline it, or a request to end their life, are embodied in the autonomy principle. Doing no harm can sometimes mean helping a

---

98   Tom L. Beauchamp and James F. Childress, *Principles of Biomedical Ethics*, 7th Edition (Oxford: Oxford University Press, 2012).

person and her family accept the inevitability of death rather than pushing for further treatment just because it is possible (nonmaleficence). When a person must make a decision for a loved one who is unable to speak for himself, they are advised to make the choices the patient would request, not necessarily the ones they themselves would want (autonomy).

For many people, ethics is rooted in religious belief. What to do and the reasons behind right and wrong are the guiding principles of all religions. Some religious groups promote having as many babies as possible as an act of faith. Decisions about treatment choices in serious illness can be influenced by faith, as well. For some, God's will means accepting death when illness presents itself. Jehovah's Witnesses, for example, refuse blood transfusions even if it means they might not survive. For others, God's will might mean that it is necessary to fight for life at all costs.

Ethical issues can start even before pregnancy. Ideally, decisions about if and when to get pregnant should be made when a woman and her supportive partner want a baby. Indeed, it should be her choice whether to be sexually active or not at any time (autonomy).

In reality, women have not always had a choice regarding when and with whom to mate. Historically, women have been bargained away to form countries, build business empires, or create the right heirs. In our times, each year, an estimated twelve million girls around the world, at less than eighteen years of age, marry against their will.[99] Government policies have an impact on reproductive rights. In the 1940s in Quebec, politicians encouraged Catholic families to have more babies to keep the balance of power with the French-speaking contingent of the province, by introducing baby bonuses. Until recently, China imposed a one-child family quota, for economic and ideological reasons.

---

99   "Child, Early and Forced Marriage," Government of Canada, last modified August 20, 2020, https://www.international.gc.ca/world-monde/issues_development-enjeux_developpement/human_rights-droits_homme/child_marriage-mariages_enfants. aspx?lang=eng. See also: "Statistics: Child Marriage around the World," UNICEF, last modified March 2020, https://www.unicef.org/stories/child-marriage-around-world.

Contraception was illegal in many countries until relatively recently and still is in some. At any rate, before the pill, birth control measures were only partially effective. Spells, incantations, herbal remedies, and numerous other treatments have been used through the ages to try to prevent unwanted pregnancies. Condoms worked, unless they broke, and only if they were used properly. Diaphragms had to be fitted the right way. But basically, if a woman had intercourse, chances were pretty good that a pregnancy would result. Women had little control over whether they would get pregnant or not. And then oral contraception was invented.

The initial introduction and testing of the pill is a tale of questionable ethics. Released in 1960, the first oral contraception pill, Enovid, was tested on unsuspecting women in Puerto Rico. It did prevent pregnancies, but it also caused irregular bleeding, depression, and a serious risk of blood clots. Present-day pills use a much lower dose but still have significant side effects and risks.[100]

The IUD was designed to prevent implantation of a fertilized egg, and so prevent pregnancy. This innovation opened up a whole other ethical question: when does a pregnancy start—when the egg is fertilized, or when it is implanted? And that question led to the question of when a fetus becomes a human, which became a legal, religious, and ethical issue.

In Canadian law, a fetus becomes a human being at the time of his birth. This law is at the core of the legality of therapeutic abortion in Canada. The law stands behind a woman's right to control her own body and her right to terminate a pregnancy. However, that does not mean everybody feels it is the right ethical choice.[101]

Abortion rights in Canada have a complicated story. Historically, Indigenous peoples used certain plants to terminate unwanted pregnancies, and settler midwives did the same. The Criminal Code

---

100   Suzanne White Junod, "FDA's Approval of the First Oral Contraceptive, Enovid," Update (July–August 1998), https://www.fda.gov/media/110456/download.

101   Abortion Rights Coalition of Canada, *Fetal Rights in Canada* (Position Paper #63) (Vancouver: Abortion Rights Coalition of Canada, October 2019), https://www.arcc-cdac.ca/wp-content/uploads/2020/06/63-fetal-rights-in-canada.pdf.

was introduced in 1892 and included a prohibition of abortion as well as the sale, distribution, and advertisement of contraceptives. Contraception and abortion "under certain circumstances" were decriminalized in 1969.[102],[103] In 1988, the Supreme Court of Canada struck down the abortion prohibition as unconstitutional and infringing on a woman's rights to her own body. The Court ruled in 1989 that a man has no right to veto a woman's abortion decision. So Canada does not have any law restricting abortion at all, and it is treated as a medical procedure controlled by the provinces. Access to the procedure is legal but limited in some areas of the country for various reasons, such as provincial differences in attitudes and implementation, as well as financial and geographical barriers. There have been a number of appeals, fights to allow or disallow private abortion clinics, petitions to overturn abortion rights, and threats and attacks against doctors who performed the procedure over the years. The present federal government has stated it will not reopen the discussion, but there is still controversy.

Roe v. Wade (1973) was a landmark decision of the U.S. Supreme Court in which the Court ruled that the Constitution of the United States protects a pregnant woman's liberty to choose to have an abortion without excessive government restriction.[104] So in the U.S. at the present time, abortion is legal in all states (although with variations in availability), and there are ongoing arguments and legal battles for and against continuing this status. At the time of this writing, a number of states in the U.S. are enacting laws restricting access to legal abortion, and a Supreme Court ruling is pending.

---

102   *The Canadian Encyclopedia*, s.v. "Abortion in Canada," by Linda Long, last modified January 15, 2021, https://www.thecanadianencyclopedia.ca/en/article/abortion.

103   "Abortion Rights: Significant Moments in Canadian History," CBC News, last modified March 27, 2017, https://www.cbc.ca/news/canada/abortion-rights-significant-moments-in-canadian-history-1.787212.

104   NCC Staff, "On This Day, the Roe v. Wade Decision," *National Constitution Center* (blog), January 22, 2022, https://constitutioncenter.org/interactive-constitution/blog/landmark-cases-roe-v-wade.

Internationally, there are ongoing political and moral discussions around abortion. In spite of a historically liberal stance, Poland has just enforced a near-total abortion ban (January 2021).[105] And at the same time, Argentina just legalized abortion in certain circumstances, although many doctors are claiming conscientious objection status.[106]

We need to remember that in the past, where legally sanctioned therapeutic abortions were prohibited, unwanted pregnancies were often dealt with in "backroom abortions," sometimes in unsafe, unsterile conditions. It would be a tragedy to see that happen again.

The ethical and legal battles around the right to die are just as complex as the abortion issue. I will address those in detail later in the chapter. But the same ethical questions apply. Does the right of the individual to decide when her life should end override the law that prohibits taking the life of a person?

Eugenics was a popular philosophy in the early twentieth century. It aimed at improving the human population through controlled breeding, decreasing "undesirables" such as the poor, the mentally ill, and certain racial groups. It was carried out by forced sterilization and by promoting birth control to certain groups. Though now recognized as a discriminatory and racist plan, it once was endorsed by governments and influential organizations and individuals. Sexual sterilization laws were repealed in the 1970s in Canada. However, between 1966 and 1976, over a thousand Indigenous women were sterilized in Canada, most often without proper consent. There are indications that this coercion was still occurring in 2021.[107] Mentally-challenged women have been subject to the same practice.

---

105 "Poland Enforces Controversial Near-Total Abortion Ban," BBC News, January 28, 2021, https://www.bbc.com/news/world-europe-55838210.

106 Daniel Politi, "Abortion Is Now Legal in Argentina, but Opponents Are Making It Hard to Get," The New York Times, March 7, 2021, https://www.nytimes.com/2021/03/07/world/americas/argentina-abortion-opposition.html.

107 Standing Senate Committee on Human Rights, Report to the Standing Senate Committee on Human Rights Forced and Coerced Sterilization of Persons in Canada, June 2021, https://sencanada.ca/content/sen/committee/432/RIDR/reports/2021-06-03_ForcedSterilization_E.pdf.

Thalidomide was first introduced as a sedative but was widely used in controlling nausea in pregnancy in the 1950s and 1960s. Fairly quickly, it was noted to be linked to many congenital abnormalities, most often babies born with missing arms and legs. The drug had been released without any testing on humans. Now there are strict guidelines on which medications are safe during pregnancy and how testing must occur. The whole area of ethical testing of treatments and medications has been influenced by the thalidomide tragedy.[108]

There are ethical issues with the testing of treatments in the terminally ill. Experimental medications might be offered in a last-ditch effort to cure or prolong life, but it is very important to be clear that this is research and that studies include placebos. Some people might opt to take part in these experimental treatments, even if they may not benefit directly, to help future generations. The principles of nonmaleficence, autonomy, and justice all have a part here.

A woman has the right to control over her own body, even during pregnancy. If she smokes or drinks, uses street drugs, or engages in other dangerous behavior, there are no laws in Canada to prevent it. But there are laws that mandate that a physician must report certain things to Child and Family Services. If there is suspicion a child is at risk, this agency has the power to remove a child from his mother's custody right after birth. The policy is under scrutiny and is being questioned or discontinued in some provinces. There are many political and systemically racist components to this mandate, such as the overzealous use of it against Indigenous mothers. There are concerns that separating children from their mothers at this early age can adversely affect infant-parent bonding. The four ethical principles all apply. The law was designed to protect children, but upon further examination, the right thing to do is far from simple.

In our society, we place great value on individual rights. But sometimes choices have to be made for the greater good. During

108   Neil Vargesson, "Thalidomide," *Reproductive and Developmental Toxicology*, no. 31 (December 2011): 395–403, https://www.researchgate.net/publication/287529627_Thalidomide.

war or disasters, when there are multiple injured people, triage procedures come into play. The person in charge of triage must make life-and-death decisions on the battlefield or disaster site and decide who gets treated first, who is beyond help and must be left untreated, and who gets into the lineup for treatment after the first group. There are protocols, but I'm sure a lot of the decision-making comes from the gut.

Triage might be an issue right now, in the middle of this COVID-19 pandemic, as demand exceeds resources for ICU beds, supplies, and vaccines in many places around the world. There will always be limited resources. There are only so many hospital beds, so many surgeons, so many operating rooms, so many ICU beds, and so many donated organs available to transplant. Time and time again, there are choices to be made about who is more deserving of life-sustaining options.

Excellent prenatal care should be available to all pregnant women. Access to proper nutrition and support for labour and delivery choices should be universal. The fact is that they are not equally available, and maternal and infant death rates are higher among Black and Indigenous communities in Canada and the U.S. The ethical principle of justice in medical care means making sure treatment resources are distributed equally, regardless of race, gender, sexual orientation, economic status, and religion, and regardless of physical or mental disability.

At the other end of life, a person has the right to accept or decline treatment for a terminal illness and the right to excellent medical care regardless of that decision. Unfortunately, many Canadians do not have access to palliative care services when they are dying, so the justice principle falls short. Helping patients decide how aggressively they wish to treat their disease and when to switch to a more palliative form of care involves the principle of autonomy as well as the goals of doing good and doing no harm.

Just as the definition of the beginning of life is controversial, the exact time of death is open to interpretation. Traditionally, death was defined as the cessation of a heartbeat. Now that breathing and the heart can be kept active by artificial means, this definition becomes problematic, and now death is largely defined as brain death. Even this way of thinking is not without controversy. When higher brain function is lost, but brain stem activity remains, the heart and lungs can continue to work. However, the person does not have awareness, and any functioning is at a basic, reflex level. Very occasionally, people in this state recover, giving the general public the impression that "brain death" can be reversible. Once there is no brain stem function, breathing and heart function cannot continue without artificial support.

It is helpful to clarify this difference so that the decision regarding stopping the machines can be made more rationally. There are ongoing ethical, legal, and religious discussions about these definitions. In Canadian law, there is actually no universal definition of death. It varies by province, ranging from a statement about irreversible cessation of brain activity to simply leaving it up to the physician on the case.

An example of an ethical and legal dilemma is seen in the case of Karen Quinlan. In 1976, at the request of her parents, U.S. courts declared that Karen could be taken off life support, allowing a natural death. At the age of twenty-one, Karen had consumed Valium and alcohol while on a crash diet. She fell into a persistent coma and was placed on life support. She remained in a coma and was shown to have some brain activity, but there was no hope that she would return to normal. Her parents successfully fought to discontinue "extraordinary means of prolonging her life," and her respirator was removed. But because the feeding tube was not believed to be causing her distress, its use was continued. Karen Quinlan died nine years later of respiratory failure.[109]

Largely because of this case, ethics committees became common in hospitals around the world, and the right-to-die movements sprung up, challenging the laws that charged a caregiver with

---

[109]   Robert D. McFadden, "Karen Ann Quinlan, 31, Dies; Focus of '76 Right to Die Case," *The New York Times*, June 12, 1985, https://www.nytimes.com/1985/06/12/nyregion/karen-ann-quinlan-31-dies-focus-of-76-right-to-die-case.html.

murder "if death was accelerated." These challenges have increased at the same time as new advances are being made to keep a body alive.

In 2017, The Supreme Court of Ontario ruled that twenty-seven-year-old Taquisha McKitty was in fact dead, rejecting arguments presented by her family that she was alive and had the right to continued mechanical life support. The court stated that someone who is brain dead "is not a person and it would be incorrect to interpret...the [Canadian Charter of Rights and Freedoms] as conferring legal personhood upon [her]." In simple terms, they stated that if a person is legally dead, it is not necessary to continue to keep their heart going artificially. Life support was withdrawn, and Taquisha McKitty died of natural causes on December 31, 2018.[110]

To quote from the *British Medical Journal*:

> Occasional stories of "miraculous recoveries" from comas are widely reported and may have led to an exaggeration of the small chances that patients have of recovering from a persistent vegetative state among a public that is increasingly well versed in this condition...

> We believe that there is confusion among the public over the differences between brain stem death and a persistent vegetative state. This, combined with high profile reporting of miraculous recoveries from coma, has led to the development of unrealistic expectations of the potential for recovery of patients who are brain dead. The confusion is further complicated by cultural and religious beliefs about death which may vary from the medical and legal definitions...

> It is important to raise the public's awareness of brain stem death and its implications. The public needs to know that by definition there is no chance of recovery from brain

---

110 Tory Hibbitt and Jonathan Rossall, "Ontario Court Leaves Definition of Death in Doctors' Hands," The Canadian Bar Association, April 1, 2019, https://www.cba.org/Sections/Health-Law/Articles/2019/Ontario-court-leaves-definition-of-death-in-doctor.

stem death, and the differences between brain death and a persistent vegetative state need to be explained. In this case we were grateful for the involvement of the family's general practitioner, and we believe that general practitioners might also benefit from having a clearer understanding of brain stem death. Sensitive and thoughtful explanations from medical and nursing staff combined with a better understanding of the nature of this condition will help grieving families cope with this difficult situation.[111]

Organ retrieval for transplant is also affected by the definition of death. Organs have to be viable to be of use for transplant, so artificial life support needs to be continued in a brain-dead person until the organs can be harvested. Legal and ethical questions around consent continue. Even with a document stating the patient's wishes, such as a signed driver's licence stating consent, a family's reluctance to allow removal of organs sometimes takes precedence. And if no prior consent is found, the next of kin are allowed to make the decision.

The Canadian Medical Protective Association (CMPA) reviewed the issue of these conflicting wishes in an article titled "Organ and Tissue Donation: Who Has the Final Say?"[112] They comment that many families who decline organ retrieval from their loved ones regret their decision. In contrast, a much smaller number of families who do donate organs feel remorse for giving permission.

To increase access to donor organs, some jurisdictions are now looking at presumed consent unless there is documentation declining permission to harvest organs from a deceased person for

111   J. M. A. Swinburn, S. M. Ali, D. J. Banerjee, and Z. P. Khan, "Ethical Dilemma: Discontinuation of Ventilation after Brain Stem Death," *The British Medical Journal* 318, no. 7200 (June 1999): 1753–1754, https://www.ncbi.nlm.nih.gov/pmc/articles/PMC1116089/pdf/1753.pdf.

112   "Organ and Tissue Donation: Who Has the Final Say?" CMPA, Advice and Publications, last modified April 2021, https://www.cmpa-acpm.ca/en/advice-publications/browse-articles/2017/organ-and-tissue-donation-who-has-the-final-say.

transplantation. Nova Scotia just passed this into law in 2020, the first of its kind in North America.

The biblical injunction against murder is echoed in basically every world religion. Until fairly recently, suicide was seen as an abomination, and assisting a person to commit suicide was seen as an act of murder. Victims of suicide were barred from religious burial. The act of suicide itself was illegal until 1972 in Canada. We now strive for a more preventive stance, with the focus on mental health promotion and the reduction of the desperation that leads a person to consider ending their life. Mental health organizations, schools, and support groups work hard to reduce the incidence of suicide, one of the leading causes of death in people between the ages of eighteen and forty-five.

At the present time, it is not illegal to commit suicide in Canada. If a person has or expects to have terrible suffering, suicide is an option. But this can be difficult, messy, and not always successful. And for many, it can be physically impossible due to the kind of suffering caused by the disease itself. As an option, some have promoted the concept that others may assist the ill person in ending their life. The decision to ask for medical assistance to help a suffering person die has become more acceptable. Ethical dilemma? Of course.

There are a number of terms used to describe this concept, with subtle but important differences.

Terminal sedation/palliative sedation is the administration of medications, usually by IV infusion, designed to decrease the level of consciousness and ease suffering but without the intention of shortening life or causing death. It is acknowledged that the person's death might occur earlier than it would without sedation, but the intent is not to hasten dying. This option is presented as an alternative to deliberately killing the person.

Euthanasia, sometimes called mercy killing, is the act of intentionally ending a life to relieve suffering. It can be active, involving actually doing something, or passive. Withdrawal of treatment is usually not classified as euthanasia, but some people argue that anything that allows for the death of an individual means you are involved in causing their death. There is an implication that it might be done without the consent of the individual.

Assisted suicide is the act of helping another person end their life at their own request.

Medical Assistance in Dying (MAiD) is the wording the Canadian Government uses to allow doctors and nurse practitioners to provide medical help to a person to die in specific circumstances. The American term used most often is *Physician Assisted Dying (PAD)*.

Please note the inherent bias in the terminology as well as a degree of overlap. The literature often uses these terms interchangeably, disregarding subtle differences in acceptance and bias.

There are a number of organizations worldwide, growing in prominence since the mid-twentieth century, which have promoted the right to choose death, some by lobbying for legal changes, and some by providing information on how to commit suicide oneself or with help. Dying with Dignity, Right to Die, the Hemlock Society, Dignitas, and Final Exit are only a few. Perhaps this trend was influenced by the autonomy and consumer rights movements that also led to changes in maternity care in the mid-twentieth century.

Long before changes in the law were contemplated in North America, some countries, such as Holland, Belgium, and Switzerland, among others, allowed doctors to provide lethal medication and offer assistance to end a life. In the U.S., a number of states have laws on the books allowing assistance to die, most notably Oregon's 2007 legislation.

The concept that a person might choose to end their life or have help doing so when their suffering becomes intolerable has been a thorny ethical as well as legal question for a long time. In Canada, the route to the present law involved a number of legal challenges. I think it will be helpful to look at the history and present legal status here in Canada.

Robert Latimer was convicted of the second-degree murder of his teenage daughter by carbon monoxide poisoning in 1993. She was severely disabled and suffered seizures and extreme pain.

Certain groups felt that this mercy killing was an act of love and should not have been punished. Others, including the courts, felt that it was not Mr. Latimer's decision to make.[113]

Sue Rodriguez was a woman with ALS who wanted permission to have others assist in ending her life, as her disabilities rendered her physically incapable of doing it herself. She could have travelled to Switzerland. Instead, she and her friends and family chose to defy the law in Canada in an attempt to force a change in the legislation. In 1994, she died by suicide with the help of undisclosed people after an unsuccessful challenge in the Supreme Court of Canada.[114]

In 2015, in Carter v. Canada, the families of Kay Carter and Gloria Taylor challenged the law against assisted suicide as contrary to the Canadian Charter of Rights and Freedoms. This challenge was successful, opening the door to the legalization of Medical Assistance in Dying (MAiD) in 2016.[115]

This bill provided a protocol for assisting a person to die if there was "a grievous and irremediable medical condition," their death was "reasonably foreseeable," there was intolerable suffering, and all other options were explored."[116] The person had to be mentally competent at the time of death, and there were many safeguards embedded into the process, including having numerous consultations with at least two healthcare providers and a mandatory delay.

An amended bill was passed in March 2021, allowing people to meet the criteria for MAiD if there was intolerable suffering,

113 *The Canadian Encyclopedia*, s.v. "Robert Latimer Case," by Edward Butts, last modified August 22, 2021, https://www.thecanadianencyclopedia.ca/en/article/robert-latimer-case.

114 *The Canadian Encyclopedia*, s.v. "Assisted Suicide in Canada: The Rodriguez Case (1993)," by Gérald A. Beaudoin, last modified November 1, 2021,https://www.thecanadianencyclopedia.ca/en/article/rodriguez-case-1993.

115 "Medical Assistance in Dying," Government of Canada, last modified August 13, 2021, https://www.canada.ca/health-canada/services/medical-assistance-dying.html.

116 *The Canadian Encyclopedia*, s.v. "Assisted Suicide in Canada," by Tabitha de Bruin, last modified February 24, 2022, https://www.thecanadianencyclopedia.ca/en/article/assisted-suicide-in-canada.

even if death was not foreseeable. It also modified the requirement that the person must be alert and able to give consent immediately before the procedure. If there is a possibility the person might not be competent by the proposed time, they are now allowed to give written consent ahead of time. Other amendments will be discussed in the future, including whether to allow MAiD for mental illness, for advance consent in the case of dementia, and for consent by minors.[117]

I am aware of at least one case in which the person's family requested pain medication be withheld so that he would be alert and competent to consent at the planned time of assisted death. It seemed a horrible conundrum, and the recent amendment would have prevented the problem. The person in question, by the way, had the sense to die on his own before the issue had to be addressed.

In Canada as well as around the world, there will clearly be an ongoing conversation as we struggle through the ethical and legal questions around assisting a person to end their life on their own terms. My comments pertain to the Canadian law as it stands today, recognizing that things will inevitably look different in the future.

Personal disclosure: Doug and I were both opposed to the law allowing medical assistance in dying when it was introduced. Doug, as a palliative care professional and as a hunter, said that killing anything changed a person, and it was too much to ask of a doctor, someone who had pledged to save life, to have to end it.

I was not happy with the law because I felt that it did not do enough to protect the vulnerable in our society. I think obvious abuses could occur, which could lead to a slippery slope and a disrespect for the rights of the disabled, the elderly, or the poor. I still have grave concerns and hope that the government treads lightly before opening up the idea of advance consent for MAiD.

---

117 "Medical Assistance in Dying," Government of Canada, last modified August 13, 2021, https://www.canada.ca/en/health-canada/services/medical-assistance-dying.html.

It is current policy in Holland to euthanize, with parental consent, newborns with severe physical abnormalities.[118] I remember a situation in my hospital years ago. A baby was delivered with severe abnormalities and was not breathing well on his own. One of the nurses insisted that resuscitative measures should be carried out, while another felt it would be kinder to just let nature take its course. I wish I could remember what was done at the time. I do know the baby did not survive.

Organizations such as People With Disabilities continue to lobby against the law in Canada, fearful that they are at risk. Bill C7, an amendment to the law on MAiD (2021),[119] again states that people must be made aware of all other options of care when contemplating MAiD. However, as a recent episode of Brian Goldman's CBC radio series *White Coat, Black Art*[120] pointed out, being aware of options and having access to them may be two different things. People with disabilities who require help with daily activities face long waiting lists and a lack of resources. Would assisted death feel like a better option?

I fear that subtle coercion is possible, and we need to be vigilant. Elder abuse is very real and could play a part. For example, a family member might suggest that a person could ask for MAiD before they run out of money for care. Or so that they "won't be a burden."

I think it is easy for an able-bodied person to think that life would not be worth living if they were paralysed or had memory loss. But I have seen, so many times, that people find joy in their lives after being confined to a wheelchair. And I have seen many of my

---

118 "Euthanasia and Newborn Infants," Government of the Netherlands, accessed March 28, 2022, www.government.nl/topics/euthanasia.

119 Bill C-7, *An Act to Amend the Criminal Code (Medical Assistance in Dying)*, First Session, Forty-Third Parliament, 2020, https://www.parl.ca/DocumentViewer/en/43-1/bill/C-7/first-reading.

120 Jonathan Ore, "Do Changes to Assisted Dying in Canada Help the Most Vulnerable or Endanger Them? Advocates Are Divided," *White Coat, Black Art*, CBC Radio, last modified March 22, 2021, https://www.cbc.ca/radio/whitecoat/do-changes-to-assisted-dying-in-canada-help-the-most-vulnerable-or-endanger-them-advocates-are-divided-1.5954154.

patients living with Alzheimer's disease enjoy the simple pleasures of a familiar face, a recognized song, or the taste of an ice cream cone. If the person had directed that "if I can no longer talk to my loved ones, I want to be put to sleep," that joy would be unfulfilled.

My other concern has to do with my beloved palliative care. At present, many Canadians with terminal illnesses do not have access to palliative care services. If it becomes easier to die by medical assistance, will good palliative care services still be promoted?

Will the incentive exist for research for curative treatments and for better end-of-life care now that the option of simply ending life is available? Will the pharmaceutical companies and scientists continue research for potentially lifesaving treatments with the same enthusiasm?

The financial cost of MAiD is lower than the cost of excellent palliative care. I would hate to think that we could kill people to save society money. (Again, here I am speaking as a Canadian, with universal health care and the costs borne by the government and taxes.) In the U.S., some jurisdictions (about ten when I last checked) have laws allowing assisted death. I wonder how many poor or marginalized Americans would choose assisted dying as their only financial option.

On the other hand, there is a possibility that underdocumented mercy killings or botched suicide attempts could increase if MAiD were not available as an option for dealing with end-of-life suffering.

Have we made it too easy to say, "Just end my life"? The time of life when a person knows death is imminent can be heartrending. But it can also be emotionally fulfilling, a time that unites families and helps people find inner strengths.

In the case of pregnancy and parenthood, things changed in terms of choice when the pill was introduced. The availability of effective birth control means couples can decide when or if they want to have children. And they often decide to wait until their finances are in order or until the woman has developed her career. More choices are now available, with advancements in fertility treatments such as IVF (in vitro fertilization).

Historically, if a woman was barren, it was God's will, and that was that. You accepted your lot (or, if you were Henry VIII, you discarded that queen and tried again with the next one). If you were blessed with eighteen children, that was God's will, too. You raised the ones who didn't die and sent them out into the world to make more children.

Having the option to die on our own terms adds another layer of complexity in decision-making. We don't get to decide whether to contract a terminal illness. But now that it is legal to ask for MAiD in Canada, the person has to make a choice. It is no longer simply God's will when a person will die. Along with decisions about treatment, a person may grapple with determining the time and place of their demise, even when they know that death is the inevitable result of their illness.

Before this possibility became a reality, I think a large number of people would have assumed they wanted this choice. They might have viewed a prolonged illness and increased dependency on others as undignified and bad. But faced with death, many people cling to life, even in reduced circumstances. It seems contradictory, but I have seen and heard it many times—an acceptance of the inevitability of death, while wanting to hold on to the preciousness of this life.

If there is the assurance of excellent pain and symptom relief, of support for the person's mental and spiritual needs, of family and loved ones' presence, and a time to reflect on life, the urgency to end life may be lessened. On the other hand, if a person knows they have the option to end their life on their own terms, that can be a comfort.

In 2017, Doug contracted a rapidly progressive form of ALS, or Lou Gehrig's disease. He lost control of his ability to speak, to swallow, and eventually even to move in his bed. All that remained was his mind and some minimal control of his hands so that he could write. He wanted to die and could not do it himself. He asked for MAiD.

The team and his physician were very good. I was impressed that they did address all the concerns I had and all of Doug's questions.

They came to our home on a number of occasions, spoke to him, and waited as he slowly wrote his thoughts down; they sometimes saw him alone, sometimes with me.

I know he struggled with the decision. The morning he planned to die, he asked me, "Am I doing the right thing?" When he asked me that question, it hit me like a ton of bricks. He had talked about—or rather written me notes about—MAiD for months. But part of him clung to life.

That moment lingers for me. I hadn't thought about how difficult it would be for him to "pull the trigger." It was not, of course, my decision. It was his. In the end, the last thing his doctor asked him was, "Are you sure you want this, Doug?" He smiled and put two thumbs up. And then died peacefully.

Was it the right choice? For him, yes. For me? I was "done," too. Exhausted, sad, aware I had already lost him. But the right thing? I can't answer that. I don't know.

Doug used to say when dealing with his palliative clients that by and large, people want life. Families get tired, want it to end. "How long can this go on?" they would ask. But a person's will and desire to live is huge, on an elemental, fundamental level. So having the right to decide to end your life does not necessarily make things easier. It can add yet another difficult choice.

As a society, are we better off having this option? Yes, in balance, I think we are. It comes down to the autonomy principle. If a person chooses, and believes that is what is best, who are we as doctors or as a society to tell her that she has to go on suffering?

There is another important ethical issue to consider. What about the caregiver? What if a doctor is opposed to abortion, but his patient requests one? Is he compelled to do the procedure? To refer her to someone who will? What if the caregiver or the pharmacist believes contraception goes against their religious beliefs?

Similarly, should a doctor, a nurse, a pharmacist, or a hospital board be compelled to provide Medical Assistance in Dying when a person meets the legal criteria? Or should they be able to opt out of something they believe to be ethically and morally wrong?

Any ethical decision must be viewed from all sides. So while I am an advocate for the freedom to choose abortion, I understand people who want to protect an unborn child. And while a person may have the right to seek help in ending their life when it is no longer tolerable, I think it is vital to protect the right of the professional who does not want to be part of an act they deem immoral, be it abortion or medical assistance in dying.

In 2019, the Court of Appeal for Ontario upheld the legality and constitutionality of a College of Physicians and Surgeons of Ontario (the medical governing and licensing body of Ontario) requirement that all doctors must provide information about MAiD or at least a referral to someone who will discuss it with the patient.[121] Physicians opposed to the requirement say that by giving the information, they are forced to be accessories to what they feel is morally wrong.

There is also the ethical and legal question about fitness to consent. At what age is a child able to understand the consequences of medical consent? This can affect choices around treatment for severe illnesses and even MAiD, as well as choices around contraception and abortion. The legal answer and the true answer are not always the same. And at what level of dementia is a person able to give consent to treat, to live, or to die?

There are many more ethical conundrums in dealing with both ends of life. Should abortion be an acceptable way of dealing with a fetus who is less than perfect? The "wrong" sex? Should people be able to say that they want MAiD if they become mentally incompetent in the future? What rights or responsibilities should a father have over an unborn child?

Of course there are still more ethical dilemmas to come. Science has a habit of providing tools to do many things before we as a

---

121   Christian Medical and Dental Society of Canada v. College of Physicians and Surgeons of Ontario, [2019] O.N.C.A. 393, https://www.ontariocourts.ca/decisions/2019/2019ONCA0393.pdf; "Medical Assistance in Dying," The College of Physicians and Surgeons of Ontario, last modified April 2021, https://www.cpso.on.ca/Physicians/Policies-Guidance/Policies/Medical-Assistance-in-Dying.

society have a chance to think ethically about the full consequences. We can harvest stem cells from aborted fetuses. Should we? We have the technology to freeze eggs, sperm, fertilized embryos. How much of a leap will it take to freeze body parts to use later, brains, whole bodies? And what could that mean for future generations?

We have extended the average life expectancy through public health and medical advances. How will that impact the earth in the future? And how old will we go? How old do we want to go?

We can keep a body alive by artificial means pretty well indefinitely. This ability was developed to reverse sudden cardiac events and as a stopgap measure until the body could heal, but as we have seen, in many cases, it has become a way of simply prolonging the dying process and taking away the very humanity we aim to preserve.

It is common knowledge that medical students swear the Hippocratic oath as they start their medical practices. The wording of this oath, written in 275 AD, does carry some universal principles, but there are parts that are no longer relevant. There are newer versions of the oath, but to be perfectly honest, I have absolutely no recall of reciting any oath on graduation. I know that I made a personal commitment to do my very best for all of my patients in all aspects of care. As I hope I have shown, decisions related to care at both ends of life are rarely straightforward. Using the framework of ethical decision-making helps navigate this minefield. It's never as simple as "just do the right thing."

CHAPTER 9

And Suddenly...

*Sadly enough, the most painful goodbyes are the ones
that are left unsaid and never explained.*

—Jonathan Harnisch

Tokothanatology: Although we strive to plan and know how to deal with the natural progress of childbirth and dying, this is not always possible in real life. Care for people faced with unexpected events can be enhanced by the study of tokothanatology. In this case, it is more likely that our knowledge of palliative care will teach us about how to handle crises in obstetrics, rather than the other way around.

THERE IS A KNOCK AT THE DOOR. A POLICEMAN IS STANDING there. He asks if you are Mrs. Smith and proceeds to tell you your husband has been in an accident. He did not survive...And suddenly, your world changes forever.

Missy lives on the street. She has gained some weight but doesn't think much of it. When she starts having terrible stomach pains, her friends finally convince her to go to the Emergency department. The nurse quickly determines Missy is pregnant, in labour, and almost fully dilated. She has had no prenatal care. And suddenly...

So far, we have looked at some of the similarities at both ends of life, and especially the care we can provide to our patients. But sometimes things happen without any warning, and there is no time to prepare for the dramatic emotional impact of these sudden events, both around childbirth and with the loss of life. Grief over the sudden loss of a loved one, whether an unborn child or a life-long partner, has a different character than the feelings associated with expected events. To help people deal with this kind of grief, it is worthwhile to understand some of the different emotions they may experience.

Everybody hopes for the perfect baby, born at term, after an easy pregnancy, a short labour, and perfect delivery. Sadly, this is not always the case. Catastrophic events happen, and pregnancies do not always go as planned. It's really quite the miracle that any babies are born perfectly, but of course most are. The steps that have to play out so that a baby is conceived, developed, and delivered are complex and fraught with challenges.

Sudden events occur in pregnancy, labour, and early child-hood. One out of four pregnancies likely results in miscarriage. Unexplained stillbirth occurs in two to five out of every thou-sand live births (twice that rate in Black women in the U.S.). In this day and age, at least in North America, maternal deaths in labour and delivery are rare, but still prevalent in certain segments of society. Here in Canada, maternal death rates in Indigenous communities are three times higher than in the white, middle-class population. Infant death rates vary around the world. The average infant death rate in Canada in 2018 was 4.8 out of every thousand live births.[122] Just to put things in perspective, in 1901, in Toronto, 167 of every thousand babies

122   "Table 13-10-0713-01: Infant Deaths and Mortality Rates, by Age Group," Statistics Canada, January 24, 2022, https://www150.statcan.gc.ca/t1/tbl1/en/tv.action?pid=1310071301.

died before their first birthday.[123] In 2001, the rate was six out
of every thousand.[124]

Infection, abruption (separation of the placenta before birth),
and other complications can cause sudden fetal distress. Going
into premature labour can leave a woman completely unprepared
and increase the risk to the child. Even a difficult delivery, the need
for an epidural, or the unplanned emergency caesarean section are
reasons for grief in some.

I dealt with many patients who lost babies at all stages of pregnancy and early childhood over the years. Grief can vary dramatically, especially in the case of a miscarriage. For a small number
of women, it is just a fact of life, a missed period, and of no great
significance. For most, though, this was a child, and the loss needs
to be grieved to a greater or lesser extent. Reaching out and supporting whatever emotions the parents (and often other family
members) are feeling is so important. When the loss is closer to
term, at the time of the birth, or shortly after, encouraging people
to arrange funerals or memorials of some sort can help with the
grieving process. Photos of the baby and memento boxes do help.
My hospital had a policy of giving a little gift to bereaved parents,
such as a sculpture of an angel with the child's name on it.

A parent may also grieve when a less-than-perfect baby is born
to them. They must grieve the loss of the expected before they can
go on with their new reality. It might take only a few seconds, or
it might go on for a long time. The parent may think of the many
"firsts" they will miss out on, the first steps, the first words, and so
on. They may feel guilt or anger, or be totally overwhelmed and
unwilling to relate to the newborn. They may face many challenges,
such as marital difficulties, pressure on other siblings to join in

123 Stacey Hallman, "An Exploration of the Effects of Pandemic Influenza on Infant
     Mortality in Toronto, 1917–1921," *Canadian Studies in Population* 39, no. 3–4 (Fall/
     Winter 2012): 35–48, DOI:10.25336/P6DW46.

124 "Health Surveillance Indicators: Infant Mortality," Toronto Public Health, August
     2017, https://www.toronto.ca/wp-content/uploads/2017/12/8c8a-tph-hsi-infant-
     mortality-2017aug18.pdf.

the caregiving, and the physical and mental demands of caring for a child with special needs.

It is useful to acknowledge all of these feelings, but also to help parents see ways of coping with their new reality. Many children with Down's syndrome, for instance, have proven to be a joy to the family. Disfiguring abnormalities or intellectual disabilities are not what parents plan for, but most find the strength to make a good life.

One of the things these parents may have to deal with are the congratulatory messages that inevitably come after the birth of a baby. The messages can come from acquaintances who are not personally involved, or from stores or companies that are aware of the pregnancy but unaware of the unexpected outcome, be it miscarriage, stillbirth, or a baby with difficulties. Being proactive and warning families that these messages may be upsetting, and perhaps even giving them some scripts on how to deal with these calls, can be helpful.

After a stillbirth:

"I'm afraid we lost our baby. It's a very sad time for us, but thank you for thinking of us."

"This is a difficult time for us. We are dealing with the loss of our child. Please take us off your call list, but thank you for reaching out."

"Just stop calling, damn it!" (I'm not recommending this one, but it is what some bereaved parents might want to say.)

With a child born with difficulties:

"Thank you" is likely all that is needed.

Some families will want to discuss the problems their child is dealing with, while others will want to take some time, and disclose issues to a chosen few. There are good sources of support, especially peer support groups, which are now available online as well as in person. Encourage parents to reach out to family and friends for support. People are often reluctant to step forward to help, not knowing what the family needs.

And where there are challenges with the newborn, letting the parents know that you will assist in the process of finding out what help is available and how to access it will go a long way in supporting them in a difficult, scary time. Most importantly, helping them to find the positive, the love they will have for this baby, no matter what struggles await them, is part of our job.

I remember delivering a baby with severe facial abnormalities and being aware that my own facial expression and my first words to the parents would have an impact on them. I took a breath, looked at this little human being that was going to have surgeries, struggles, turmoil his whole life. I saw kicking legs, felt a strong heartbeat, and heard a robust cry. "Your baby looks strong," I said. "He is beautiful and healthy. There are some things that will have to be dealt with, and I will help you through this. As you can see, he has some problems with the way his face came together, but you can see all the parts are there. We will get what he needs."

And we did. He had a quick cuddle with his parents before being transferred by ambulance to a neonatal unit in the city, and had his first surgery within hours of his birth. A feeding tube allowed him to get his mother's pumped breast milk along with other sustenance. He has had numerous surgeries and has done well in life. I hope the first words I said to the parents gave them some strength for the struggles they faced over the years. I wish I could say I did as well in every case, but of course I learned through experience what worked and what didn't.

We need to balance empathy with professionalism and offer the support and answers the parents need. Shared tears can be powerful and helpful; offering sound advice and plans, equally so.

One of my first recollections of this kind of experience was early in my practice. My patient had had a perfectly normal, easy pregnancy, was near term, and presented to my office just a little bit worried. She hadn't felt the baby move for a few days. While fetuses do sleep, they do not go more than a few hours without activity.

We regularly suggest kick counts to be aware of the baby's movement, and a simple check of the heartbeat is all that is needed to reassure the mom. But this time, there was no heartbeat. Doppler:

nothing. Over to the hospital for an ultrasound: no heartbeat, no movement. For some unknown reason, this baby had simply died.

When we observe a sudden change in the fetal heartbeat, an emergency caesarean section can sometimes save the life of the baby. But in this case, there had been many hours and perhaps days with no activity, and there was no hope for this child's survival.

Rather than a futile surgery, these parents elected to deliver naturally, or almost. When there is no life, the hormones which initiate labour often do not rise, so we induced labour and delivered a beautiful but lifeless baby. I tried hard to make it as normal a delivery as I could and allowed the parents to hold the baby and say hello and goodbye. It is common now, but in those early days of my practice, this was not the way we dealt with stillbirths. The baby would have been delivered as expeditiously as possible, whisked away, and the mother shuffled off to a surgical wing of the hospital so as not to upset the other mothers. A few years later, I heard from these parents, who now had a healthy newborn baby. They wanted me to know the way I had helped them with the loss of their first child had made all the difference to them.

After a catastrophic event, telling the truth in simple, understandable terms is vital to help people understand what happened, and why. This is especially true when there is a question of human error.

I was involved in a delivery where a drug error occurred, and a long-acting narcotic was given to a woman in labour instead of the usual short-acting one, causing the mother to be very drowsy, and her baby to have difficulty breathing after birth. We were able to reverse the drug effect in the newborn with a simple injection, and the mother recovered without difficulty, although she missed out on remembering the delivery. Later, I sat down with the parents and explained what had happened and how the error had occurred. I promised that new protocols would be put in place so that a similar error could not occur again. The couple appreciated the honesty and were reassured there would be no long-lasting consequences.

In another case, we had a perfect delivery, done by a medical student under my supervision. But the baby did not pink up well.

We gave oxygen, naloxone (a medication to reverse the effects of narcotics), supported respirations, and so forth, but could see no improvement. After discussing with the pediatrician, we transferred the baby to the city by ambulance. The pediatrician soon called me and said this baby was dying, but the cause was not clear. We were able to get the parents to the city by ambulance so they could be with him as he died.

An autopsy showed heart abnormalities not compatible with life. The baby had thrived during the pregnancy because his oxygen was provided through the placenta, but his own system could not function by itself.

The student who had delivered this baby and I did a housecall to tell the parents the results of the autopsy. We sat at their kitchen table with the parents and their five-year-old daughter and explained what the postmortem had revealed. The little girl said, "So my baby didn't get any blood to his brain, so he died and went to heaven. I understand." I'm tearing up writing about this all these years later. My student was so moved by this experience, she went on to specialize in obstetrics.

Someone (well, Doug) pointed out to me that I reacted the most strongly with loss and struggles surrounding childbirth. Even as I'm writing these stories now, I feel the heartbreak, the sadness, the loss. People deal with sudden events around childbirth similarly to any traumatic situation. They need to come to terms with the reality and then deal with their new world.

Everybody hopes for a peaceful death, in old age, surrounded by loved ones, after a fruitful and satisfying life. And if not that kind of death, at least one in which you have time to say goodbye to loved ones, to review your life and deeds well done. But it doesn't always happen that way.

While heart problems, cancer, and other diseases cause the most deaths per year globally, accidents, injuries, and overdoses still account for a significant number of deaths around the world. And just because someone dies of heart disease doesn't mean they die slowly. Disease can strike suddenly and progress quickly, sometimes within minutes or even seconds. Sudden death is possible in the healthy and the chronically ill alike.

Death by suicide places an extra burden on the surviving family and friends. When a person takes his own life, family members and friends have to deal with another layer of complexity in their grief and require a different kind of support. They have to deal with the what-ifs, the guilt of not recognizing the person's pain. As caregivers, we have the goal of helping a grieving person heal and come to terms with the loss. And of course, part of the family physician's role is to deal with mental illness and address suicidal thoughts before tragedy strikes.

Doug was called to many suicide cases in the community over the years. He talked about helping the families with their grief, but even more so about the needs of the first responders and the trauma they had to process. Supporting and acknowledging the burden caregivers and first responders deal with on a regular basis as part of their jobs can go a long way toward easing PTSD symptoms in these individuals.

Similarly, with homicide and with accidental death, whether motor vehicle accident, work-related, or accident at home, there is no preparing, no chance to say goodbye. Helping the survivors come to terms with this loss can be challenging.

Many people live with chronic illnesses or expect to have a long course of their illness before they succumb. But sudden death can occur here, too. For instance, a person with MS may die suddenly from a heart attack. The grief process for survivors takes on a different tone. They have lived with a heightened awareness that this person will die but can be taken completely unawares just the same.

I worked with a mother struggling after the sudden death of a child who had a chronic debilitating illness. Helping her realize that her feelings were the same as if the child had not had his underlying disease allowed her to move forward with her grief.

While it may seem that palliative care plays no role in unexpected deaths, many of the principles can be applied to supporting the loved ones left behind in these "sudden" situations. The support needed is complicated by the shock of the death. There was no time to plan, no time to say goodbye. The grief process may be difficult, especially where there is unfinished business—a fight, an argument, a discussion not yet completed.

Professionals involved in these crises feel the impact, as well. Recognizing this and working together to debrief is a valuable exercise. Acknowledging our own feelings is as important as helping our patients. And taking time for self-care, especially when it seems there isn't time to do so, is essential.

Deaths sometimes occur in large numbers. Here in Canada, natural disasters often seem far away. When the news announces 230,000 dead in a tsunami in Indonesia, or 300 dead from an earthquake in Italy, it seems distant and unreal, unless, of course, we know somebody directly involved. It is human nature, I guess, to feel just a bit of sympathy but no real involvement when something occurs on the other side of the globe. War, natural disasters, mass shootings, and perhaps in the near future, deaths due to climate change are unfortunately part of the human experience. We grieve collectively as well as individually.

As I write this, we are in the midst of a pandemic. Millions of people are infected with the virus all around the world. Thousands of people have died of COVID-19 in Canada, millions worldwide, and the numbers are still rising. The whole world is in lockdown. We are not able to be with loved ones in long-term care facilities, and many are dying without family or familiar faces around them. Mental health challenges are at unprecedented numbers, as the fear and the social isolation, along with economic hardship, take their toll. Social isolation means that weddings, funerals, and other gatherings are taking place virtually or not at all. Funerals are different now. A friend of mine died just as everything was locked down. The planned funeral was postponed and then cancelled. His widow is philosophical about it. But she did not have that chance to mourn with friends and family. As the world reels with the shock of so many deaths, women get pregnant, babies are born. The circle of life goes on, even during a pandemic.

An oncologist told me how difficult it is now to give bad news, from six feet away rather than next to a person with a hand resting on their patient's forearm or shoulder, and often without the support of a loved one in the room.

The principle behind social distancing is to "flatten the curve" so that hospital resources aren't overwhelmed with cases requiring intensive care and respirators. This pandemic has put the ethical principle of justice to the test. What about the cancer patient who happens to get sick during this crisis? Or the child with a broken arm?

Healthcare and frontline workers have borne the brunt of the extra work and the risk of exposure to the disease in order to care for their patients. The emotional toll of being in that position is easy to understand but hard to live with. A lot of the decisions about how to deal with all of this are made by governments and health provision agencies. The day-to-day reality for frontline workers is the patient in front of them, and what can be done for this individual at this particular time. I think the way to survive as a healthcare provider is just that: one-on-one with the person who needs something you have to offer, whether it is a procedure, a medication, or simply a kind, caring glance.

With any sudden death, the "patient" is the one left behind. While the same emotions described for a dying person are mimicked in any grief reaction, these feelings may be less accessible or more volatile after a sudden death. There is no time to come to terms with the impending death. There is no ability to say goodbye, to deal with unfinished arguments, unfinished business. And often wills and finances are in the usual disarray of "we will get around to that someday."

Sudden, unexpected events happen. Our role as caregivers is the same as it is in any of our encounters with people at both ends of life. The principles of family-centred maternity care and of palliative care can help you guide your patients through the difficult times. Sometimes the only thing we can do is "walk alongside."

CHAPTER 10

Lessons Learned

Nobody cares how much you know, until they know how much you care.
—Theodore Roosevelt

How people die remains in the memory of those who live on.
—Dame Cicely Saunders

Tokothanatology: When it comes right down to it, the main thing in caring for people, especially as they live through the major transitions at both ends of life, is good communication. To listen—to share thoughts and information in a meaningful, compassionate way—is the essence of good tokothanatology. Sharing in the joys and trials of childbirth was a wonderful part of my general practice. I found the same kind of satisfaction working with my patients at the other end of their life cycle.

IN THE FIELD OF TOKOTHANATOLOGY, I'M NO EXPERT. I HAVE never given birth; I have never died. The real experts have always been my patients. I learned so much from them. I'd like to share some of these insights with you now. Take from them what you will. I hope they will make practicing tokothanatology a little bit easier and a lot more satisfying. These are the gentler sides of caregiving, the things I didn't necessarily learn in school but rather by experience.

Over the years, we have learned in the field of obstetrics that involving our patients in the process of birth provides a better experience for all involved. This is just as true in end-of-life care. Yes, there are many ways that people die, and yes, the circumstances are much more variable than in pregnancy and childbirth. Still, if we look at dying as a process just like giving birth, we can provide excellent care and a more fulfilling experience for the dying person and her family.

I know there are family doctors who shy away from providing palliative care. There are many reasons they refer patients who need this care to the oncologists and the palliative care teams. They cite lack of time and lack of skill along with the emotional toll of this aspect of medical care. We don't have to do all that the specialists do. We don't have to have knowledge of the most up-to-date chemotherapeutic advances. But by keeping a connection with these patients and their families, we fill a huge gap in care.

Many family doctors don't do deliveries, either, but they have an ongoing relationship with the pregnant woman, and then the newborn along with the whole family. So, too, with the dying person. Even if you refer out all of your patients who have terminal illnesses, you will still be involved with them in some way, and you will still be involved with their families.

I have to admit my bias here. I believe that primary caregivers provide the best longitudinal care to patients and their families. I used to say my practice was "pre-cradle to post-grave." I know that doesn't happen everywhere, and it is less common than it used to be. But whether actively doing obstetrics and palliative care or not, the role of the family doctor is vital, in my opinion. We see the whole person, not just the disease.

One of the joys of being in general practice for a long time in a small community was the relationship I had with multiple generations of a family. I took care of a number of four- and five-generation families over the years. One family I can think of involved a single mother of a teenage girl. This girl became pregnant, and the woman planned to help raise the baby so her daughter could continue school. While the daughter was in labour, the woman's father was admitted to hospital in end-stage heart failure. Fortunately, it was a small hospital, so she was able to go back and forth between her loved ones. Physically, this back-and-forth may have been easy, but it was certainly a challenging emotional time for her. She was able to be there when the baby was born, and she was able to be with her father when mom and baby were brought over to visit with him. He died later that night.

I cared for another family over many years, a great-grandmother, a grandmother, and her four daughters. Later, I delivered a number of the daughters' children, and some of their children—five generations! I also cared for the rest of the grandparents and all the spouses. The great-grandmother moved in with the family of one of her granddaughters, where I provided palliative care for her. She always said I was one of "her girls." I would sometimes get the names and the generations mixed up in my head, as you can imagine.

As a family doctor, I had many roles. Quite aside from the obvious, providing the medical care, I think I was primarily a teacher. Sometimes a nurturer, sometimes a coach, sometimes a parent, sometimes a salesperson. Along the way, I learned many lessons myself.

I learned about the value of good communication. I learned it is important to give information accurately and kindly. I learned how to be honest and direct without being blunt. I learned how vital it is to repeat and to get feedback to know the patient understands. I gained skills in active listening, the art of attentive hearing, reflecting and responding to what a person is saying. I learned a lot about understanding my patient's body language. And about my own. Facing the computer screen instead of my patient, for instance, gave a pretty clear message that I was not engaging fully with them, and they knew that.

I learned to try never to use jargon. It sneaks in. Terms we use regularly may feel normal to the medical professionals but not be completely understood by anyone else. Speaking in plain language assures that our patients can understand what we are saying.

I learned that it's very important to have knowledge about medication and treatment at your fingertips but also to be able to say, "I don't know, but I'll find out for you." We don't have all the answers. We don't even know all of the questions. But as physicians, we know a lot. And our patients, for better or worse, see us as experts. So act like one. Not a god, but a teacher. I also learned how much power I had as a physician. I could convince a person of almost anything that I thought was right if I wasn't careful to balance that with alternative ideas.

I learned about how fundamental honesty is and how difficult it is sometimes. "I can see in your eyes, I'm not going to get better; don't bullshit me." But white lies can be part of the therapeutic relationship. Sometimes a person just needs some kindness, or a family to be told their loved one had a peaceful death.

Another example was my "rule of seventeens." Many of my patients during labour would ask me, "How many more pushes?" Now that I'm retired, I can reveal the secret of my answer. I always said seventeen. Always. And it always seemed to help. You see, seventeen is a number that is difficult to concentrate on when you are actively pushing, a very intense activity to be sure. But not so high that it is discouraging. Hope is a major component of staying the course, of being able to push through exhaustion and discouragement, to see the end in sight. I never did actually count how many babies were born on the seventeenth push, but at least a few were. To all the other mothers I cared for out there, I tricked you, and I'm sorry.

A lot of people fear that they are not being told the truth about their illness or that their families are being told something different than they are. I often talked to my patients with family members present so they knew they were hearing the same thing. Some patients wanted to hear things alone, to have time to digest the information before involving others. Respect for that privacy is of prime importance. I used to ask which they preferred.

In labour, as in palliative care settings, one of the common things I heard was, "You're not telling me everything." An assurance that "I promise you I will not keep any information from you" came out of my mouth many times, sometimes to the point of showing them the letter I sent off to the specialist. Actually that was a useful trick—a good referral letter should have a good summary of the illness, so going over it with the patient and family is a way of confirming accuracy and providing a written summary for them to keep and review.

I found teaching my patients how to talk to other doctors very helpful. Seeing a new doctor such as a surgeon or an oncologist can be intimidating. Patients forget what they planned to ask or don't want to appear stupid, or they just get overwhelmed. I would suggest they take someone along with them if at all possible. "Four ears are better than two." I would recommend that they write out the questions ahead of time, and write notes during the consultation or immediately afterward. One of my patients taught me a neat trick: he typed out a summary of his history and his questions and made two copies, one for himself and one for the doctor. I loved that idea.

I would suggest: ask the specialist, "What will happen if I have the surgery, and what will happen if I don't have it?" Ask them about side effects of chemotherapy, how you will feel at the time, in a week, a month, a year. Ask them about wait times, ask them how many trips you will be taking to the city. Ask them—and this is something you may or may not get an answer to, but it's worthwhile to try—"If this were you/your mother/your son, what would you do?"

Later, I would review the letter I received back from the specialist with my patient. Studies show that the information retained by a patient after a consultation with a doctor is pretty poor. In fact, 40–80 percent of information provided by healthcare practitioners is forgotten immediately. The more information, the less the retention. And when you factor in the stress of having a serious illness or a bad prognosis, the amount of information lost or misheard is even higher. According to the NIH (National Institutes of Health), patients tend to focus on diagnosis information and not on instructions for treatment.[125] So I would try to explain in clearer language what they had heard in the doctor's office and clarify the next steps.

"Listen to your patient; he is telling you the diagnosis." This was what the great physician William Osler taught his students in the late nineteenth century. I learned that people usually knew more about themselves and their loved ones than I did. When a woman says the baby is coming *now*, it likely is. I learned to take it seriously if a parent said there was something different or wrong with their child. They are the experts on their children. We are experts on disease. There's a difference. That's not to say that we should believe everything our patients self-diagnose after reading about their symptoms on Google. But when you get past that, and really listen, your patient will tell you what's wrong.

I know at least one surgeon who cancelled a procedure when the patient said they thought they would die during the operation. He felt the foreboding carried significance, and he was not alone in this.

People often have an innate sense of their own bodies. If a person says they feel an impending doom and will die soon, they just might. Some people even think that a dying person has some control over the timing. They might wait to die until a loved one comes to see them, or they might wait to die until they are alone. I'm not sure if I believe this, but plenty of people do. There are many stories about loved ones who gave the dying person permission to go. Other stories tell of a patient who held on just until a wedding, or the birth of a new baby, or the arrival of a family member from abroad. Of course, when that doesn't happen, it can be hard to accept. Doug used to say to families, "Don't feel guilty if you weren't there at the moment of death. The important times were the times you *were* there."

And I learned that allowing some of my feelings to be part of a conversation could be supportive, but that people looked to me

---

125   Roy P. C. Kessels, "Patients' Memory for Medical Information," *Journal of the Royal Society of Medicine* 96, no. 5 (May 2003): 219–222, https://www.ncbi.nlm.nih.gov/pmc/articles/PMC539473/.

mostly for strength. There is a balance between clinical distance and clinical empathy. Emotional support, the ability to reach our patients in an empathetic way, is as vital as having medical knowledge; I could argue maybe even more so. A few seconds of simply caring goes a long way, and that is what people remember. Dr. Brian Goldman, host of the CBC radio series *White Coat, Black Art*, wrote a book called *The Power of Kindness* (2018).[126] The stories he told showed incidents of kindness and empathy for others that I found very moving. I have to admit I cried most of the way through this book. He described his search for empathic people, to find out if he had lost some of his own empathy working as an emergency room doctor for many years. He came to the conclusion that although he had toughened up a bit through the years, he was still able to feel empathy.

Caring for the dying involves soul-searching on the part of the physician. Certain aphorisms come to mind; sometimes they present a better and more concise way of saying something than a long-winded discourse could.

"Cure sometimes; care always."

"Don't just do something; sit there!"

"They don't care what you know if they don't know that you care."

"You make a living by what you get; you make a life by what you give."

Part of the job of a caregiver is to confront their own emotions, to face their own mortality and that of their loved ones. When a child is ill or in danger, nurses and doctors often think *I need to go home and hug my kids*. Doing some work on ourselves, acknowledging our own mortality, is hard but vital to being an effective caregiver. But we must remember to tell ourselves: It's not my baby. It's not my death. It's not my husband.

That is one of the things I had to learn myself. If I was too distant and clinical, it appeared that I lacked empathy for the person. Although I might do exactly the right thing clinically, I

---

126 Brian Goldman, *The Power of Kindness: Why Empathy Is Essential in Everyday Life* (Toronto: HarperCollins Canada, 2018).

wasn't helping my patient as much. On the other hand, if I felt too deeply, it became about me, not them, and I lost effectiveness. People aren't stupid. They know when we are faking our feelings. They know when we are so upset we're not making good clinical decisions. And they know when we are being honest.

Samuel Shem wrote a novel, *The House of God*,[127] that I think most medical students are advised to read at some point. He talks about how people enter medical school starry-eyed, empathetic, and idealistic; but end up jaded, cold, and unfeeling. He described a list of rules on surviving medical training, which includes some pretty cynical descriptions of medical people.

The most important rule I took away from the book is that "At a cardiac arrest, the first procedure is to take your own pulse."[128] I take this to mean there is value in self-awareness and self-care. It took a number of years for me to understand this lesson, that my own needs were equally valuable. By preaching it often to my patients and my students, I think I finally embraced the concept myself.

Sometimes I felt angry, sad, overwhelmed, afraid, and not up to the task. I had to recognize my own feelings before I could be there for my patients. Accepting and acknowledging my own emotional frailty was very hard. I'm a professional; I'm tough; I have to be in charge...Sometimes taking a moment for myself before tackling the next case was all that I needed. Sometimes self-care meant really getting away, to the cottage, or at least to a complicated sci-fi-fantasy novel. Then I could step back in, refreshed and renewed.

Self-care can also mean accepting that you have to talk to a professional. There is a strong sense that as physicians, we know what to do for our patients and so should be able to figure things out for ourselves. What is it they say about a doctor who treats himself? He has a fool for a doctor, and a fool for a patient.

---

127 Samuel Shem, The House of God (New York: Bantam Dell, 2003).

128 Samuel Shem, The House of God (New York: Bantam Dell, 2003), 40, 177, and 381.

Self-care can also mean seeking out and providing support for each other. I remember one difficult case. Well, I actually don't remember the particular patient...But I remember the nurse who spent time with me in the hall after the death, recognizing my pain and supporting me, touching my shoulder, just being there. Thank you, Mary.

I learned that sometimes people can talk to each other better when there's a neutral third party present. Offering to be present when a person tells family about a bad prognosis or when there are unresolved conflicts can be extremely helpful.

Many women, in the most intense part of their labour, say some pretty awful things to their partners. "You are never going to touch me again!" "You did this to me!" "I'm never having sex again!" Those of us who have attended many deliveries have heard this kind of thing numerous times and are able to reassure their men that it is quite normal, and not to take it personally.

In the dying person, brain metastases or metabolic imbalances can cause personality changes and angry outbursts just as dementia does. They can be very upsetting to family and caregivers, so extra support and explanation may be needed. It can be very difficult not to take these episodes personally, but recognizing the anger as part of the illness can help. Otherwise, people may be pushed away inadvertently when they are most needed.

Even when a dying person is mentally clear, things they say can carry a lot of emotional weight. They may extract a promise from loved ones to do something or care for someone after they die. When a promise is made, the aftermath can be very difficult emotionally because there is no one left to compromise or discuss things with.

I learned that sometimes the family's needs had to override the wishes of the dying person. A patient in the hospital may wish to die at home. But his wife is frightened of the physical work that would be required, not sure she is up to the task. Or she might be afraid of living on in the house where her husband dies. A person may say they do not want a funeral, perhaps thinking to spare the family. Many times Doug and I would encourage families to arrange a funeral or a memorial service in spite of these wishes, without feeling any guilt. These ceremonies are really for the living—a time to say goodbye and share memories with friends and family.

When a person is dying, they may extract a promise such as "look after your mother," wanting the assurance that a spouse or a child will be cared for after they die. This may be promised with all good intentions; however, it might not be realistic or feasible. I know there are women who gave up plans for marriage to stay home and care for an aged parent. And men who took over family businesses instead of following their own career plans. And vice-versa, too.

I am aware of a young married couple who took on the care of an autistic brother because the husband promised his mother they would before she died. His wife had the difficult task of becoming the caregiver to this severely disabled man, while the husband went off to work. In this case, the marriage was on the brink of collapse until they were encouraged to place the brother in an excellent institution, pay for his care, and visit frequently. They found this was a way to honour the promise without causing damage to their own lives.

The family physician is sometimes in the position to help a loved one reevaluate such promises and come to terms with finding ways of keeping the nature of the promise without harm to themselves or others.

To quote Barbara Karnes, a hospice pioneer and blogger in Vancouver:

Promises [are] made in the sadness, fear and uncertainty of the moment. Promises we feel bound to keep because they are the last interaction we had with someone we were close to or in some cases, not so close to. Death seems to hold us hostage to the words of the moment.

I don't think we are bound to those promises. We need to look at the promises made, evaluate them as to: can it be done, should it be done, and am I willing to do it? I think the paramount principle underlying the promise needs to be how will the outcome of the promise affect the living?[129]

A few other lessons come to mind.

Along the way, I learned the importance of gaining skills for talking about difficult topics, talking about death, and giving bad news compassionately. Robert Buckman's book *How To Break Bad News: A Guide for Health Care Professionals*[130] is an excellent resource for this, along with a video series called *Communication Skills in Clinical Practice* released in the 1990s[131] on the same topic.

Sometimes, when a person says they don't want to talk, they really don't. Not saying much, but just listening, just being present, is often all someone needs. I learned that doing nothing can be just the right thing to do. Labour takes a long time, but sometimes trying to interfere causes more harm than good. Continuing treatment of cancer or other diseases can mean prolonging the dying process rather than adding to life.

Sometimes, it is necessary to be tough, telling a woman in labour she has to deal with the pain, and that to push through it or to breathe is the only thing she can do. Sometimes, acknowledging that "having a terminal illness sucks" is the only right thing to say.

And sometimes sensitive decisions must be made about treatment for cancer or other serious illness. If the patient is in a state of denial, they may not be able or willing to discuss or understand the choices offered. A bit of tough reality may be necessary to make sure they understand what "doing nothing" might mean. In my experience, patients are quite capable of discussing these hard choices

---

129   Barbara Karnes, "Deathbed Promises," *BK Books* (blog), October 18, 2017, https://bkbooks.com/blogs/something-to-think-about/deathbed-promises.

130   Robert Buckman, *How To Break Bad News: A Guide for Health Care Professionals* (Toronto: University of Toronto Press, 1992).

131   *Communication Skills in Clinical Practice* (Toronto: HEAT Inc. Health Education & Training, 1999), DVD, 71 mins.

with clarity and then going back to a stance that there is nothing wrong with them at all.

Control around pregnancy and birth and when a person is seriously ill tends to be in the hands of the professionals. For a few generations, the decision-making over childbirth was controlled entirely by science and medicine. Now we take the woman's input as a vital part of the process. Once a person becomes a patient, particularly with a terminal illness, she will commonly experience a similar loss of control. Where she used to be in charge of her own life, becoming a "good patient" can mean turning over her decision-making process to the experts.

In the hospital, all decisions about basic things, from what to wear to when to wake up, are taken away. Even without hospitalization, people often have a sense of their lives being turned over to others, to professionals as well as to loved ones. They feel unsure and vulnerable. For families, a battle for control of decision-making is common, which is why clear family conversations and advance directives are so helpful.

During labour and delivery, so much of what is happening in a woman's body is beyond her control. Having the right people there to support her is key to making the experience as positive as possible. A doula, for example, can be such a support person. A doula is a nonmedical professional trained to take on the role of the voice of the woman and her partner. She acts as an advocate and an ongoing presence during the course of labour and even afterward.

Death doulas, or end-of-life doulas, are becoming more commonly used in palliative care. Trained in ways much like childbirth doulas, they can be an ongoing support and guide for the dying person. He or she is someone who is totally there for the comfort of the patient, not to provide treatment or physical care. While I have not worked with doulas personally, I see the value of having someone present who is not actively providing medical care. A patient will often be more willing to share their concerns with someone who is not perceived to have power over them; they might be unwilling to complain to a doctor or nurse for fear of having pain medication withheld, or fear of offending and not getting the attention they want. A doula can act as a guide for the woman in labour or for the dying patient, and as a bridge between medical personnel and the patient. In some ways, Doug's palliative care volunteers acted in a similar role.

We all desire a sense of control in our lives. A woman's body takes over completely when she is giving birth. Contractions come unbidden. Pushing sensations are overwhelming. The focus of family-centred maternity care is to encourage the woman to have a say in such things as pain control, birth position, and so on. In addition, being able to decide some of the smaller things, such as what music is playing and what she wears, may be a way to maintain some semblance of order. Reassuring a pregnant woman that she has the strength, the knowledge, and the support to deal with her upcoming labour can go a long way.

In the same way, I learned from my dying patients that small things can really matter. Knowing that you have a disease that is likely going to be the way you die, you realize what is truly significant: family, spiritual awareness, and so on. But the placement of a box of tissues or the temperature of your dinner plate takes on importance just as such small details can to a woman in labour. These are things that can be controlled. At both ends of life, people tend to focus on what is immediately in front of them, and not the big world outside.

One of the things my patients taught me is to always find a way to provide hope. "When faced with uncertainty, there is nothing wrong with hope," O. Carl Simonton said.

I think that "there is nothing more we can do" is one of the most destructive things we can say. There is always something we can do. It may be looking at quality of life instead of a cure. It may be exploring whether home or hospice is the next step. Patients need to be reassured they will not be abandoned. I used to hold my hands out in front of me and swivel in my chair as I was saying that—body language—and say that we are no longer going to focus on a cure that isn't possible. *We will focus on making whatever time you have left as good as it possibly can be.*

Instead of saying there is nothing more to do, it might be better to say, "Chemo would have diminishing returns, and the side effects would outweigh the benefits, so let's focus on your comfort." This wording gives the same information but holds on to hope. A different hope, but hope nonetheless. "All is lost" is different from "Hope for a good day today." Hope your nephew comes to visit this afternoon, hope the coffee is hot enough. Or even hope that the end comes soon.

Everybody needs a sense of having value. It is disheartening for a person to feel they have no purpose in life, that they are just waiting to die. We can encourage friends and family to keep the dying person in the loop, requesting their opinions, asking advice. This time can also be used to contemplate past achievements and to reach out and connect in a meaningful way with loved ones.

I have heard many people say the period of time that they knew they were dying was the best time in their life. And some family members say they learned so much about the dying person in their last few days or weeks. They express gratitude for the gift of something more to remember the person by.

A wife of a dying man told me he had been gruff, demanding, and unreachable for years. As his health failed and he became more dependent on her, he was able to tell her how much he had always loved her, and all the things he had admired about her. He never apologized, but they found joy in those final months.

A little girl, dying of leukemia, asked Doug if he would be her boyfriend, because she wasn't going to grow up to have a real one. He promised her he would and that I would be ok with it. I have a picture of the two of them together. He was kissing her cheek as she smiled beautifully. Years later, at Doug's funeral, her father told me how much Doug had meant to her and to the family. They planned to name a special trail in the woods in Doug's honour.

We have learned over time how important it is to communicate with our pregnant patients. I think we still do rather poorly talking about death and end-of-life plans generally. If we could increase the comfort level around discussions about a person's wishes before there is a crisis, we could prevent anxiety, misunderstanding—and likely a lot of unwanted intervention. To quote Dr. Angelo Volandes in his book *The Conversation: A Revolutionary Plan for End-of-Life Care,* "Without this open conversation about death, patients are traumatized needlessly, leaving their families with the emotional scars of witnessing the hyper-medicalized deaths of their loved ones."[132]

There are ways to have this discussion before a person is actively dying. Doctors could have conversations with patients about their wishes and plans as a routine part of checkups. Another good time to have this discussion is whenever a person is admitted to the hospital for any reason. Doing this regularly normalizes the topic and gives people time to think about how they feel.

If a patient broached their end-of-life wishes in any way, I made it a priority. I also tried to have a meaningful discussion on the subject with as many of my patients as I could. Time restraints were my excuse for not covering the subject with all of them.

For an older patient, or for anyone who brought up the subject, I might say:

I would like to know your thoughts about what you would like to tell me if you were ever in a situation where you could not talk for yourself. This is not for now; I'm not saying anything is wrong with you at all. But if you were in an accident, or you had a stroke and couldn't talk, knowing how you feel would help me know how much treatment you would want or not want. This could help your family, too, so rather than guessing or fighting about it, they could follow your wishes. I will write up our discussion in my chart and give you a copy so you can share it with your family, and I suggest you keep it in your wallet, as well. I promise you it would only be used if you couldn't speak for yourself.

132   Angelo E. Volandes, *The Conversation: A Revolutionary Plan for End-of-Life Care* (New York: Bloomsbury, 2015), 4.

So, for instance, if you had a stroke and couldn't talk, and then you got a bad pneumonia, would you want to be treated, or just kept comfortable? If you had a heart attack, would you want to have resuscitation? For example, would you want us to zap your heart to get it started again?

This discussion would of course be geared to the individual's situation. For a younger, healthy person, it might be simply something like: "I would like to document your wishes for care if something drastic were to happen to you and you were not able to communicate. Do you have any special wishes? For instance, is there any surgery or treatment you would not want us to do?"

A surprising number of my older patients were quite clear that they did not want any heroic treatments. "If it's my time, let me go" were words I heard many times. Some, however, were very clear they would want all that medical science had to offer.

While having this conversation, I would stress that in any crisis situation, we would always talk to the patient first, and this documented set of requests would only be addressed if he or she wasn't able to answer for themselves at the time.

An excellent website called *theconversationproject.org* offers tools for families to have this kind of discussion.

Hospitals and nursing homes require a discussion and documentation about a person's wishes when people are facing potentially life-threatening situations. Some facilities are now including this as a standard question at the time of any admission. If it became more widespread, it might take some of the fear factor out of the practice and avoid comments such as, "Does that mean I'm dying? I'm just here to get my gallbladder out!"

Living wills, also called healthcare directives or advance directives, are documents that state a person's wishes surrounding healthcare, especially end-of-life care. Depending on where you reside, a living will may or may not carry any legal weight. But it certainly carries a moral value, outlining a person's wishes to their family and to the caregivers.

Usually the document designates a person who is charged with speaking for the writer if they become unable to communicate. The person must decide based on the writer's expressed wishes, and if there is doubt that this is being done, a hospital ethics committee might be asked to assess the situation.[133]

"Do not resuscitate" (DNR) orders are common in hospitals and long-term care facilities for palliative patients. These orders give direction to avoid heroic measures if a person's heart or breathing stops. In Ontario, there is a legal document available called a Do Not Resuscitate Confirmation Form. This form can be kept at home. (It's usually kept on the fridge; paramedics are trained to look there.)

Dr. Willie Molloy, a geriatrician in Hamilton, Ontario, first published a pamphlet called *Let Me Decide* in 1989 and later a book by the same name.[134] It is a template for writing an advance directive with good, clear explanations and examples. He encourages people to think about and write out their wishes in an "If...then..." format.

"If I can't communicate with my family, do not do any heroic treatment."

"If I cannot eat, I would like to be fed by artificial means."

"If I do not have a reasonable chance of an independent life, do not resuscitate me if my heart stops."

I found this template a very useful tool as an introduction to the subject with my patients. I would send them home with a copy of the pamphlet and offer to go through it with them if they would like, or simply let them do the exercise on their own. (I checked on Amazon.ca—the book is still available.)

This tool or others like it could be a part of a person's medical record, with the promise that it would be reviewed regularly and could be changed at any time. If a record existed of the patient's wishes, families and medical practitioners would have a much easier time deciding when to intervene and when not to.

---

133 "Healthcare Directives: What You Really Need to Know," CMPA, Advice and Publications, last modified December 2021, https://www.cmpa-acpm.ca/en/advice-publications/browse-articles/2017/healthcare-directives-what-you-really-need-to-know.

134 William Molloy, *Let Me Decide* (Toronto: Penguin Books Canada, 1992).

In reality, this discussion most often takes place in a crisis situation. The patient and her family are asked to make snap decisions about truly life-and-death matters. It would be so much better if adult children could have meaningful discussions with their parents about their hopes and wishes, from long-term care to what to do and how to deal with a life-threatening illness.

These days, most children and many adults have no experience with death as a part of life. We could expose children early on in life to the concepts of death and growing old, at home and as part of the regular school curriculum. There are many excellent books for children dealing with death and loss. And while I think of it, about childbirth too. I had a bookshelf full of them in my office to lend out.

We already have books about pregnancy and childbirth, such as What to Expect When You're Expecting,[135] Six Practical Lessons for an Easier Childbirth,[136] or The Complete Book of Pregnancy and Childbirth.[137] I look forward to a day when we have comparable books for those facing the last stage of life. Maybe I'll have to write one myself.

I learned over my years in practice that birth and death are what make a person's life real. Birth and death are universal. Yet each birth and each death is unique. A new baby brings life; a death leaves emptiness and sadness. But the way we care for our patients during these times has a huge effect on their well-being. The skills we use and the attitudes we have at both ends of life share many common threads.

---

135   Heidi Murkoff, *What to Expect When You're Expecting* (New York: Workman Publishing Company, 1984).

136   Elisabeth Bing, *Six Practical Lessons for an Easier Childbirth* (New York: Bantam, 1967).

137   Sheila Kitzinger, *The Complete Book of Pregnancy and Childbirth* (London: Dorling Kindersley, Ltd., 1980).

Conclusion

To everything there is a season, and a time to every purpose under heaven.
A time to be born, and a time to die.
A time to kill, and a time to heal; a time to break down, and a time to build up.
A time to weep, and a time to laugh; a time to mourn, and a time to dance.
—Ecclesiastes 3:1–4

There is no cure for birth nor death save to enjoy the interval.
—George Santayana

LIFE IS BOOKENDED BY BIRTH AND BY DEATH. AS A FAMILY doctor, I have had the task and the joy of providing healthcare for many people in this "interval" over my forty-plus years in practice. The greatest challenges and the greatest rewards for me have been at the very beginnings and the very ends of these lives.

I vicariously experienced the miracle of birth many times over in helping to provide a safe, satisfying pregnancy, labour, and birth. I learned clinical expertise, patience, empathy, listening skills, the whole gamut of good medical practice. Doing obstetrics made me a better practitioner and a better human being. So, too, working with people through the minefield of illness, dying, death, and bereavement called on me to learn skills, to use all my patience, empathy, and humanity in order to care for my patients through this stage of life.

In this book, I have talked about how we view birth and death and how this has influenced the practice of medicine. As physicians as well as other caregivers, we have an obligation to help as we can and to offer our presence and our humanity. But it is also our privilege to walk along this journey with our patients, to intervene when it is appropriate, or to stand by when that is the right thing to do. We have our own rules, our rituals, our best practices. We are constantly striving to improve our methods and practices to achieve the best outcomes.

Scientific advances and evidence-based medicine will continue to improve the quality of care we are able to provide for our patients at all stages of life. But we should never leave our humanity at the door. Empathy and emotional support are what people need from us and what they remember and are thankful for.

Science itself will and should question our assumptions on the best care, learning and moderating as we go, involving society, ethical considerations, personal rights, and choices.

At the same time, consumers of healthcare will and should continue to take a critical look at the rituals we call medical care, and question their value and validity.

Birth has evolved from "just what happens" to medicalization, to the backlash of natural childbirth, then back to more intervention, back and forth.

And as more people take control over what happens as they grow old, as they become ill and die, expectations change. The goals of prolonging life, curing disease, and reducing pain and suffering are good goals. We have made huge strides in improving lifespan and curing infections, cancers, and heart disease. Technological advances often provoke a backlash, both in the medical community and in society in general. Applying new science to everybody at the end of life can be hugely expensive, counterproductive, futile, and inhumane.

The pendulum is swinging toward a more muted level—pulling out all the stops when appropriate, but supporting and allowing natural death to take its rightful place.

Palliative care, hospice, death with dignity: all these consumer-driven ideas endeavor to reclaim the humanity of end-of-life care, to accept death as a normal part of life and family.

We will continue to work to cure cancer, diabetes, heart disease, ALS, and other diseases that cause suffering and death. But we will need to remember that death is a reality, and it has its beauty and its value.

I was struck early in my practice by how I dealt with birthing and dying in such similar ways. My goal has been to show you how to use this knowledge to help your patients and ultimately yourself at the beginning and end of life, as well as the middle—life itself.

My own life has been enriched by my ability to share in the lives of so many, especially as they bring new life into the world and say goodbye at the end of it.

I hope that by understanding the shared experiences, the continuity of care in obstetrics and end-of-life care, you will be able to support your patients and their loved ones and share in that richness along the way.

Acknowledgments

THIS BOOK HAS BEEN IN MY HEAD FOR MANY YEARS, BUT IT took a pandemic to make me sit in front of my computer and put my fingers on the keys. A lucky internet search brought me to Scribe Media and their online course, *The Scribe Method: The Best Way to Write and Publish Your Nonfiction Book*. By following their method, I'm able to say, "I did it!"

A sincere thank you to all of the Scribe Media staff whom I had the privilege of meeting and working with. To the members of my Guided Authors' group, thank you for all of your interest and support. I have made many friends and learned so much!

There aren't enough words to thank my editor, Jane Enkin, for the comprehensive and thoughtful editing, hand-holding, and support you gave as I was sorting out my ideas and getting them organized and coherent. You questioned and pushed me. You made me work harder and clearer, and in so doing, made this a much better book. Thank you, Janie.

Thank you to Patty Dietz, who laughed and cried with me as she listened to my "read it aloud" edit, all while she was taking care of my house, my dog Kitt, and me.

A number of people read through my manuscript, at various stages of editing, and provided excellent feedback. I appreciate all your comments and encouraging words. Particularly, thank you to Jo Owens, Lori Messer, and Taryl Felhaber for your thoughtful advice.

Thanks to my mother, Eleanor Enkin, for helping me know I could do anything I set my mind to, as long as I was willing to work for it. And to my father, Murray Enkin, for his early influence on my choice of career path, his iconoclastic attitude that encouraged me to fight for what was right and necessary, and his belief in writing it down. And thanks to my husband, Doug, who taught me that dying people are still very much alive and worthy of excellent care and support.

I would also like to acknowledge Justin Jaron Lewis, who provided helpful commentary on religious and ethical issues; and Eva Bild, doula, doula educator, and childbirth advocate, for her warm and knowledgeable insights. Thank you to my siblings Nomi Kaston, Jane Enkin, and Randy Enkin, and to your spouses, for your enthusiasm and encouragement.

There are many doctors, nurses, doulas, and other care providers who have cared for people at both ends of life, sometimes at the same time, or at different stages of their careers. Thank you for the work you do.

Most of all, I would like to thank my patients over the past many years. I thank them for allowing me to walk with them on their journeys of giving birth, raising their families, and holding the hands of their loved ones in their last days. I learned from the infants I held in my hands as they came into this world, and the people who confided in me and taught me about strength and fear, vulnerability, and faith in their last days. They truly were my teachers and the people I strived to touch in some small way to make their lives, their birthing, and their dying just a little bit better.

Author's Note

I HAVE BEEN COLLECTING IDEAS AND INFORMATION ABOUT BIRTH, death, and tokothanatology for many years and from many sources. In my home office, there is a whole filing cabinet full of notes, and a collection of ideas in the Evernote app on my phone. I had an extensive collection of textbooks and journals about obstetrical care, palliative care, and ethics, most of which I have given away. I utilized Google searches extensively, both to glean ideas and to fact-check in the writing of this book, and I do have a list of the sites I researched. I have chosen not to provide a complete bibliography in this publication but have tried to provide sources for numbers and factual information throughout. Please feel free to fact-check, as all of this material is readily available online. I have also credited any direct quotes in the text of this book. Any errors in this book are my own.